THE BOY NEXT DOOR

This is the story about how an ordinary boy who was faced with a terminal illness became extraordinary and captured my heart.

BY PEGGY LINDGREN

ISBN# 978-1-7345477-1-9

Contact Information
writebyme@yahoo.com

Edited by Nicole DeKasha
Photo Enhancement by Donald Bersano
Cover design by Alison Mitchell

~ FORWARD ~

Born in 1987, Mark Staehely was a normal, energetic, mischievous twelve-year-old boy, the star pitcher on his baseball team. He lived with his parents, Sue and Ray, and older brother Mike in a typical Midwest neighborhood. Everyone got along; it was a good life. Good, that was, until everything fell apart. Weeks of pain in his leg led to a dreaded cancer diagnosis: Neuroblastoma.

Peggy Lindgren, one of his neighbors and close friends, has written this story, "The Boy Next Door." She has carefully crafted the events of Mark's short life into a book you cannot put down. Peggy spent years writing this story. She read Mark's journals, researched the disease, and interviewed many people.

Wise beyond his years, Mark left an impact on everyone he met. His legacy lives on forever with "Make Your Mark: The Mark Staehely Pediatric Cancer Foundation."

Before retiring from teaching, I had contact with many children. After I read this story, I wished Mark had been one of them. I felt the love and joy this young boy brought to our world. I want to thank Peggy Lindgren for writing this beautiful story of such a remarkable boy.

Anne Anderson
Author and Friend

~ TABLE OF CONTENTS ~

To all those committing their lives to finding a
cure for cancer.
To the doctors and nurses caring for these
children.
To those children battling to live another day. To
all the parents fighting to keep their child alive. To
Mark, for showing us that with faith and
perseverance there will always be
HOPE

~ Introduction ~

*"I think it's good to pray because after I
pray I just feel good. First of all you
could talk to god and tell him to try and
help people who could be sick. Second of
all sometimes people have hard times
and you could talk to god and ask him
to help you. Last of all you could pray
for your family."*

Mark Staehely

It has been ten years. Ten years since my
neighbor, my friend, Mark Staehely, passed away.
Mark was only eighteen years old. Diagnosed at
age twelve with cancer, Mark was a remarkable
child who taught those around him about living,
about giving back. How does a kid dealing with a
devastating diagnosis live his life for what he can
leave behind? This is someone you should know.
This is Mark, the boy next door.

I recently retired from a job I loved for over
forty years as an office manager for a busy dental
practice. I met hundreds of people over those years
who helped shape the person I am today. I believe
the many relationships we have throughout our
lives teach us what is most important on this
journey. My relationship with Mark was one of
those that especially influenced me.

Soon after retirement, my husband and I
converted our guest room into an office/study for
me. I now had a place to call my own, a quiet place
where I could write. I arranged my desk under a
window that faces south and allows the sunshine
to enter as I begin my day. As I look out my
window, it's only fitting I can see Mark's house.

I began writing his story shortly after he died, and then life, as it so often does, got in my way. I stopped writing. Many years passed. I blamed it on many things. But Mark's story has always been on my mind. Because it has never left my heart, it is time for the story to be on paper so that others can get to know Mark and be touched by his incredible legacy.

I once shared my passion for writing with Mark, and he knew I wanted to tell his story. He told me he didn't think there was anything to say about him. He honestly had no idea the impact he would have on those who knew him—as well as the many people who never had a chance to meet him.

I have had many conversations with Sue and Ray, Mark's parents, through the years. Knowing I had started this book, they came over one morning with a large plastic bin full of articles written about Mark and several of his journals. As I sat on the floor of my office pouring over page after page, I was overwhelmed with emotion. I had grieved Mark ten years earlier, but at that moment, it became even more important to me to remember this young boy.

So, this is that story. It's about Mark, how he lived, and how he died. It is about how he made a difference to me and others. The special relationship we shared would be one that managed to touch my heart and break it at the same time. He honestly had that kind of impact on people. I saw firsthand that people didn't have to know Mark to be touched by his passion. You only have to hear his story, and he will find a way into your heart. I will share a few of these stories with you.

Chapter One: Mark

"Dear God, will you please help all the people who aren't as fortunate as me. Help all the Homeless people, starving people, people who have no one to talk to, or people that have lost their families. Make them strong and keep your hands on them. Thank you, God, Thank you for all your blessings. Amen."

Mark Staehely

Mark, a typical twelve-year-old boy, was living an ordinary, pre-teen life. He loved baseball, riding bikes, and collecting baseball and football cards. He had a passion for drawing and sketching and often gave his artwork as gifts.

Born on December 7th, 1987, Mark's favorite number became seven, and he wore it proudly on his baseball jersey, year after year.

He was small in stature for his age, but that didn't stop him from being athletic with a strong and confident demeanor. Some would even say he was a bit of a bully, but once you got to know him, that edginess was just part of his charm.

Mark Staehely.

He was headstrong and extremely stubborn. Unlike his older brother Michael, who was easygoing and cooperative, he was a challenge for his mom and dad from day one.

He had a soft spot for the underdog, possibly because of his small build. He made up for it with his energetic and outgoing personality. He was comfortable talking to people, even strangers he encountered standing in the checkout line at the grocery store. He could engage a perfect stranger and start a conversation, ending it by telling them to have a good day.

Mark came from a good family. His parents, Ray and Sue, were hardworking. Sue worked part-time at Gloria Jean's Coffees, and Ray worked at Caterpillar Tractor. His brother Michael was five years older, and Mark looked up to him.

Many people were drawn to Mark and could not explain why. He could unintentionally draw you into his world, thereby leaving his "mark" on you.

Mark was outgoing and compassionate. As a young boy, he always wanted his mom to give money to homeless people standing on the corner. One day, they were stopped at a red light, and there was a homeless man with a cardboard sign that read "Need Money." Mark insisted Sue give him something. She said, "Mark, I only have five dollars in my wallet for the week, and we need gas."

His reply was, "So, that is more than he has, and you never know if he is an angel put there to watch over us; we will be fine."

She handed over the five-dollar bill.

As if one of those angels heard Mark's plea, an unexpected gas card turned up in their mailbox a few weeks later.

Mark's smile was one of the first things you noticed about him. When he was first learning to walk, he began to run, always on the go and moving forward. Out on the front sidewalk with mom and dad surrounding him, Mark took off. He fell flat on his face and knocked out his brand new two front teeth! His permanent teeth came in a bit awkwardly, but his smile was one you could not ignore or ever forget. His adorable, huge smile got him out of many mischievous situations with his mom. Mark loved mimicking Sue's deep booming voice; it was impossible not to laugh! His mimicry was not always the most appropriately timed, but none the less he managed to get your attention.

Mark was tough, spunky, and competitive, and he loved to test his mom's patience. If the truth is told, Mark was simply a pain in the ass. Both his mom and dad would be the first to admit this fact. Those who knew him would agree, and yet somehow, he was endearing at the same time!

These traits would prove to be necessary, as he was in for the fight of his life.

Chapter Two: The Neighborhood

"I believe everyone has angels with
them all the time. You can always
talk to them and tell them all your
feelings and thoughts, they will
make you feel better. Angels are
special to me, and I feel like I have
my own angels on my shoulders all
the time."

Mark Staehely

We live in a small town, Shorewood, IL, about an hour southwest of Chicago. After searching for a neighborhood with young families and good schools, we felt we found the perfect place. Within the block, there were plenty of kids of all ages, and our two sons always had playmates.

Shorewood is an average Midwestern town with friendly neighbors. We would often wave to one or another as we drove past their houses, knowing where we could borrow a cup of sugar or a yard tool if necessary. Everyone looked out for each other, and shortly after moving in, we all formed a Neighborhood Watch program. We even had a few block parties over the years. Overall, it was a safe and happy place to call home.

The Staehely family lived next door. Michael was preparing for high-school graduation and had been accepted to Illinois State University. Mark had just finished sixth grade.

Our families didn't have coffee in the morning or cook burgers on the grill on weekends. We were simply neighbors with boys close in age, and we enjoyed the overall feel of this neighborhood.

Mark's best childhood friend was JP, who lived directly across the street. JP and Mark had been best friends since moving to the neighborhood as toddlers and were the same age. Mark either liked you, or he didn't. He was often a total clown and the center of attention. He enjoyed playing in a group or was content being alone with his sports card collection. He liked to flirt and joke around, and everyone appreciated his crazy sense of humor.

My earliest memory of Mark came when the boys were old enough to play outside together. At about five and six years old, the boys were running around between our houses, being typical boys. I heard some commotion and walked around the corner to find Mark with his shirt up. There was a bite mark on his back, and Alex, our youngest son, was standing there, eyes down, shoulders sagging. I immediately walked the boys over to Mark's house and rang the doorbell; Sue came to the door. She looked at the bite and said to me, "It happens. Let them work it out."

She was not angry or annoyed. I turned to Alex and asked him what he had to say, and he looked at Mark and said, "I'm sorry." The boys continued to play as if nothing had happened. This incident was a great lesson in tolerance and forgiveness for both Alex and me.

Yes, our families were neighbors, and because of Mark, we would soon become friends.

CHAPTER THREE: THE RED FLAGS

*"Dear God, I want to tell you that I'm
going to be writing prayers and
asking you for things. Help me
please to feel better and stronger
each day. Finally Please watch over
me and my family. Thank you for all
your blessings."*

Mark Staehely

As parents, we spend every waking minute
worrying about our children. We take them to the
doctor for all the necessary well-baby check-ups
and immunizations. We worry when they sneeze
and cut that first tooth. We do everything we can
to keep them safe from harm, from covering all the
electric outlets to putting baby gates up by the
stairs. We bandage their skinned knees, comfort
them when they are sick, and pick them up when
they fall down. We know when something is
bothering them long before they will even admit to
it. There is not a single thing we would not do to
keep our kids happy and safe.

Spring 2000

The first warm day of spring, Mark was out
bouncing on the new trampoline he had gotten for
Christmas. The trampoline was a huge attraction
for all the neighborhood kids. It was not unusual
for the kids to be out there for hours, jumping and
having a typical play day.

Later that day, Mark began complaining of
leg pain. Sometimes only one leg would bother
him, and other times they would both hurt. He had
not fallen or injured himself that he could

remember. He was a rough and tough kid, not one to complain, especially if it meant he had to stay inside and not run around to play.

Sue and Ray decided no more trampoline for a few days to see if maybe he had strained a muscle. The leg pain continued. The first of many red flags went up.

Mark's parents didn't consider it a huge concern; however, it became apparent that something was wrong. Mark was not a complainer, so Sue, to be on the safe side, made an appointment for him to see his pediatrician. The doctor could not find anything wrong and sent him home suggesting Ibuprofen.

After a couple of weeks, Mark continued to complain. Sue noticed a slight limp, so she made another appointment. On this visit, the doctor said Mark was having "growing pains" and would be fine. Several weeks later, after numerous appointments, the pediatrician told Mark to run down the hallway in his office. Mark did as he was told. The pediatrician looked at him and said, "See Mark, you can run. Now go out and play."

Frustrated that nothing had improved or been resolved, Sue and Ray took Mark in for yet another office visit, and the doctor suggested Mark needed a consultation with a psychiatrist. At this point, desperate for any answers for his constant pain, be it mental or physical, they followed up and made an appointment. The consultation proved that there was nothing mentally wrong with Mark. He was not depressed or looking for attention as implied.

Dismissed...They felt as if they had been dismissed. The worry and frustration continued.

Mark was 12 years old, weighing only 56 pounds.

Mark may have been small in stature, but he was tough and athletic. He made up for his size with determination and attitude. He was a competitive boy and worked hard to be the best he could be. Because of his passion for the sport, his baseball coaches couldn't help but notice him. He had a strong arm and was the starting pitcher for his Little League team.

He loved watching baseball and studying the game. His skills were sharp, and his head was always in the game.

One Saturday morning, a couple of weeks after his visit to the psychiatrist, Mark suddenly did not want to go to his baseball game. This was a boy who lived for baseball and was an All-Star player. His parents encouraged him to go and play his game. The game began, and Mark was the leadoff hitter. He walked up to the plate, put the bat on his shoulder, and just stood there. Mark was unable to swing the bat. He had no strength at all. He simply put the bat down, walked over to his mom and dad, and said, "I want to go home."

That would be the final red flag because Mark loved playing baseball. There was nothing he enjoyed more. Sue and Ray drove him home. The rest of the weekend consumed them with worry.

The following Monday, Sue was back on the phone with the doctor; she was not going to rest until she had some answers. She refused to take Mark in for another wasted appointment and insisted on a referral to an orthopedic doctor. Sue wanted to be sure he did not have a bad sprain or a broken bone. X-rays were taken. Once the orthopedic doctor read the x-rays, he ordered an immediate bone scan. The doctor referred Mark to a specialist. Something was seriously wrong.

No one can imagine the worry and anguish Ray and Sue were going through. Their worst nightmare was happening.

Mark had known his pain was real all along.

CHAPTER FOUR: FROM NEIGHBORS TO FRIENDS

"Dear God, Please give me the strength and power to do things with my family and friends. Please be with me when I go to the hospital. Also please bless all my Doctors and nurses. Please bless my Mom who is always there for me. And please watch over everyone who needs help. Thank you for all your blessings. I love you. Amen."

Mark Staehely

It was a warm evening, Friday, June 16, 2000. We were leaving early the next morning for our family vacation, and I was upstairs packing. I heard the doorbell ring, as I had many times before. It was an odd time of night for visitors, and my back stiffened. Suddenly, I had an uneasy feeling in my stomach, like the one you get when your phone rings in the middle of the night. I stopped folding clothes and strained to listen when my husband, Dave, answered the door. When I heard the tone of his voice calling me, I knew my intuition was right.

He immediately called me downstairs. "Peggy, Sue is here." It was apparent to him; this was not a casual 'I need to borrow a cup of sugar' visit.

My mind was racing, and my heart was pounding as I quickly walked downstairs. It was a visit I had been dreading for weeks, and deep in my gut, there was a feeling of profound uneasiness.

"Mark is sick, really sick," she said. Sue's eyes were glazed over, and her voice shook with nerves. She needed to borrow a suitcase, she said. "We don't even own a suitcase; we never go anywhere."

I invited her in, ran upstairs, and frantically pulled my clothes out of the bag I had been packing. I felt a sudden rush of panic and overwhelming dread. Words were not forming in my head.

As neighbors, we had all been aware of Mark's struggles and the many doctor appointments. It had been a couple of weeks since the trampoline had come down and since we had seen him running around the neighborhood. We'd shared an unspoken worry. Now that worry had become a bitter reality.

I ran downstairs and set the suitcase at her feet. I reached out my arms, and we hugged without words. I felt a fierce connection with Sue at that moment: we were no longer just neighbors; we were friends. Because of Mark, we became forever changed. I would reflect on this encounter for many years. For Sue and me, it was the beginning of a lifelong friendship. There is something both compelling and unique about the mom connection. As we stood in the doorway, mom to mom, she didn't say much more. She didn't need to.

Cancer: A word no parents should ever hear, much less comprehend, and should never, ever have to explain to their child.

The doctor had suggested they gather loved ones together and prepare for the hospital. After a couple of hours and a few phone calls, their home filled with family and friends. This support would surround and sustain them for a journey they did not want to take.

CHAPTER FIVE: THE DIAGNOSIS

*"Dear God, I need to ask you for a few
more things, first of all I need help with
my new medicine. Please help me take
my medicine well, also please direct my
medicine to go to the bad stuff and
destroy it forever. Last, please help me
do good with this medicine so all other
people can have it help them to. Thank
you for all your blessings. Amen."*

Mark Staehely

Neuroblastoma. According to the Mayo Clinic, it's "a rare childhood cancer, [that] most commonly affects children age 5 or younger, though it may rarely occur in older children. In 2 out of 3 cases by the time it is diagnosed it has already traveled to the lymph nodes or other parts of the body. It is rarely found in children older than ten years.

Neuroblastoma most commonly arises in and around the adrenal glands, which have similar origins to nerve cells and sit atop the kidneys. However, neuroblastoma can also develop in other areas of the abdomen and in the chest, neck and near the spine, where groups of nerve cells exist.

Neuroblastoma begins in neuroblasts, immature nerve cells that a fetus makes as part of its development process. These nerve cells are found in several areas of the body.

As the fetus matures, neuroblasts eventually turn into nerve cells and fibers and the cells that make up the adrenal glands. Most neuroblasts mature by birth, though a small number of immature neuroblasts can be found in newborns. In most cases, these neuroblasts mature or disappear. Others, however, form a tumor, a Neuroblastoma.

It occurs slightly more often in males."

They found a tumor on Mark's adrenal gland. There will always be a question as to how long Mark may have had this tumor. Was his low weight and small build an indicator of something going wrong in his body? No one had ever suggested this as a concern.

Mark was in Stage IV, meaning it had metastasized to distant lymph nodes, bone marrow, liver, skin, or other organs. Mark was considered to be high risk, due to his age, weight, and raging hormones. The diagnosis terrified them, and at that time, doctors were unable to give them a prognosis.

CHAPTER SIX: THE JOURNEY BEGINS

*"Dear god, will you please watch over
me while I'm having my surgery. Help
me to be strong and not afraid because
I know you and my angels are always
with me. I love you lord, thank you for
all my blessings. Amen."*

*"Dear god, I'm very thankful of all the
things you have done for me. Please
make me stronger everyday, and
healthier get all this bad stuff out of my
body and help me when I'm in the
hospital not to get sick. Thank you for
all my blessings. Amen."*

Mark Staehely

Mark understood something serious was
going on because he couldn't remember the last
time he wasn't hurting. He was not a child, but
then again, he was far from being an adult. Mark
knew he was very sick as he sensed the urgency of
the hospital admission and the frantic look on the
faces surrounding him. Mark was relieved to know
something was finally going to be done to help him
feel better, but he had many more questions that
he didn't know how to ask.

Sue and Ray needed to process the
diagnosis and decide the best way to approach the
subject with Mark. During these first few days,
they were very cautious not to use the word
"cancer."

A cancer diagnosis is difficult for an adult to
wrap his or her head around; how do you tell your
child he has cancer? They explained to Mark that
he had this "bad stuff" in his belly, and he would
need surgery to have it removed. They were

advised to keep the explanation simple, and as Mark asked questions, they could address them one at a time.

The doctor referred Mark to a specialist at a hospital near Chicago. He was admitted, poked, prodded, x-rayed, and scanned. The next day they performed a painful bone biopsy, and although he had been given a twilight anesthesia, he was acutely aware of the procedure and, unfortunately, he remembered it.

Mark would need surgery to remove the tumor the testing had revealed on his adrenal gland. He met his surgeon, and they immediately bonded. Mark told her right away about what had happened during his biopsy and that he had not been asleep. He was aware of everything happening around him. She assured him that would never happen again!

On the day of surgery, she stopped in to see Mark. The doctor sat down on the bed next to him and promised she was going to do everything possible to remove the "bad stuff" in his belly. Suddenly overwhelmed with emotion, Mark's surgeon began weeping, tears running down her cheeks.

Embarrassed by her sudden display of emotion, she slowly turned around and looked at Sue and Ray. "I am so sorry. I never cry."

Mark gently took her hand and said, "It's okay; I trust you."

The doctor took Sue and Ray out into the hallway and said to them, "I cannot explain that outburst, and I apologize again. He touched my heart so profoundly, and I find myself drawn to him." Sue and Ray understood. They had heard this comment many times over the past week from many others who were caring for him.

The surgery was expected to last approximately four hours. In the waiting room, about forty people gathered together to support Sue, Ray, and Michael. Most people were standing and pacing. Others offered to bring food in for the group. Four hours came and went. Finally, a nurse came out to update them and explained it was taking longer than anticipated. It would be another three hours before the doctor came out to a waiting room full of family and friends.

She told them Mark was doing well, his vitals were normal, and he was in recovery. She explained his tumor had "spidered" out, and the surgery was more difficult than she first expected. She told them it had little fingers that moved outside the adrenal gland, up towards his esophagus, and back into his spinal column. It had been a very delicate procedure.

After hearing this report, Sue looked at the surgeon and said, "Okay, but did you get it all?"

She responded, "Yes, Mrs. Staehely, I did. Every single bit."

Another hour passed, and Mark woke up in recovery, groggy and medicated. Sue, Ray, and Michael were by his side. Mark sleepily looked up at Ray, and the first words he mumbled were, "Dad, can I get a four-wheeler?" Without 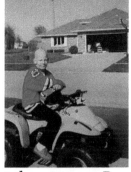 hesitation or a second thought at the expense, Ray said, "Sure." In reality, Ray knew they couldn't afford one, but at that moment, that didn't matter.

What mattered was the look on Mark's face when he said yes. For Ray, that look was worth anything. He bought the four-wheeler. He felt that if it gave Mark something to look forward to and get excited about, he would worry about the cost later. And let's face it, Mark knew that timing was everything!

The protocol for Mark would be months of chemotherapy and radiation. It would include hospital stays and many outpatient visits.

One day, Mark's aunt was visiting, and they were alone in his hospital room. He had been thinking about everything and decided she would be the best person to approach with an aching question. "Do I have cancer?" He had known only older people who had cancer. She immediately turned and left the room. She explained to Sue and Ray what Mark had asked, and she did not feel she could be the one to tell him.

It wasn't necessary. Mark knew the answer. He may have wanted to hear the truth, but deep down he already knew.

They continued to refer to his illness as the "bad stuff." Ray clearly remembers it would be a year and a half before they spoke the word "cancer" to Mark.

This was just the beginning of their journey.

CHAPTER SEVEN: MARK'S OWN WORDS

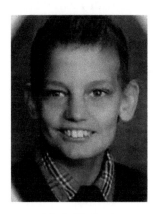

Mark 6th Grade

*"Dear God, I want to tell you that I'm
going to be writing prayers and stuff
in my journals and will be asking
you for things. Help me please to feel
better and stronger each day.
Finally Please watch over me and
my family. Thank you for all your
blessings. Amen."*

Mark Staehely

Mark loved to write. He kept several
journals over the six years of his illness and wrote
many prayers, often several a day. He wrote of
feelings he was unable to express verbally.
Sometimes he would date them, but usually he
would not.

He also had several sketch pads, and he
would spend hours drawing and creating artwork.

Among Mark's possessions that Sue and
Ray shared with me were these journals. I found
many loose-leaf pages folded neatly in his books.
As I sat in my office and looked through the poems

and prayers that he had hand-written, I came across this paper. While fortunately many of his prayers, poems, and artwork are available for me to share, this writing was the only one I would find in which Mark expressed his first thoughts. He wrote of how he felt those first few days. Mark wrote this when he was fourteen years old, two years after his diagnosis.

Mark lived his faith every day, as is clear in his prayers and his actions. I feel it's important to share his writings precisely as they were written. Pardon and embrace the grammar and misspelled words.

"I'm gonna tell you a story about a young man. That young man is me. My name is Mark Staehely, I am 14 years old. I have 1 brother, his name is Michael, My moms name is Susan and my Dads name is Raymond. Im gonna tell you a story that started June 16th 2000, that day changed my family, my friends and life forever. That day was a nightmare. I was diagnosed with a rare disease called Neuroblastoma, that is a childhood form of Cancer. The doctor that day took my Parents into the lunch room of Hope hospital and told them the bad news. The doctor said I could stay over night or come back in the morning. So we went home that night and my mom called everyone. Before I knew, there were 30 people over at my house.

I was very afraid of the words "CANCER" and "TUMOR", if somebody said either of those words I would get afraid and upset. I thought of cancer and I thought of not living. So...the next morning we went back to the hospital and got admitted. I was in for 2 weeks, those 2 weeks I had gotten my surgery and chemotherapy. I was very scared about getting surgery but I had all my family there to help me. And I also knew that if would help me to get better and survive. The only thing I can rember about going to surgery is seeing my cousins Matt and Colleen, they gave me hugs before entering to get surgery. We had an angel surgen that went in and cut the tumor out and it was very successful. She got all the tumor out and nothing went wrong. The tumor was located on my andreanalin gland. After that I was very sick and out of it. But I still got through it with help of my family and friends. After surgery I had to get chemotherapy to kill all the cancer throughout my body. After 2 and a half weeks in the hospital I finally got to go home. When I got home all I wanted to do was see my friends, and I couldn't because my blood counts were down and I was in risk of infection. At hope hospital there were 2 doctors, they were both really nice. And of course the nurses were great, I had about 12 nurses and I loved all of them. But I had a special 2. There names were Jenny and Laura. They were probally in there late 20's. They were angels. So after we got home we had to back twice a week, so we did that for 2 weeks and then I got admitted into the hospital for chemotherapy. So we kept rotating 2 weeks off and then in for a week or so. We did that for 4 months. We met a lot

*of great people there and they took good
care of me. But we all thought because it
was time for my stem cell transplants we
would go to Children's Memorial hospital in
Chicago. My Uncle had called a few days
before that and made an appointment with
a doctor. So a few days later we left hope
and started new at Childrens Memorial
hospital. I was very scared about the whole
idea, but when I got there I knew it was a
great place and that's where I needed to be.
So when we got to CMH we met my doctor
and the first thing he said was he's to small
and doesn't weigh enough. So then he
started me total Prerental nutrition (we
called it TPN) and thank god he did that or
else I don't think I would be doing good at
all. I was on that stuff for 9 months. And
when I started I weighed 57.5 pounds and
today just over 2 years I weigh 77.5 pounds.
I gained 10 pounds a year just on TPN. I had
a lot of precidures done on me why I was
going on chemotherapy. One terrible
memory was when I had to have a
bonemarrow biopsy, that's when they take a
long needle and dig in your backbone and
get marrow out. Marrow is wat ur blood
counts r in. (Red, white, and platelets) Well
my doctor tried to put me asleep and he
thought I was out cold but I wasn't and he
went ahead and did it."*

Mark's protocol was aggressive
chemotherapy and eventually radiation. Also, the
discussion for stem cell transplants began. He

would stay in the hospital for many weeks during these treatments.

Mark was an ideal patient. He loved his nurses and doctors and did everything they asked of him. Mark made a habit of asking them how they were before they had a chance to ask him how he was feeling, a most unusual way for a young patient to greet the staff, but it immediately endeared him to them. The nurses would rotate their schedules so each of them could share in his care.

He surprised and amazed his mom and dad with his positive attitude and his willingness to cooperate.

And then everything changed.

CHAPTER EIGHT: THE MOVE

*"Dear God, I've been feeling alone lately
and I'm kinda sad. Can You lift my
spirits, and also keep me strong because
I got things to do in my life. Please help
everyone who is sad and depressed.
Last keep watch over my family and
friends. Thank You for all my
blessings."*

Mark Staehely

A few days after surgery, Mark was able to go home. He was thrilled to be leaving the hospital but dreading the next phase of his treatment. The doctors wanted him to rest and gain some strength before he would begin his chemotherapy. Friends were allowed to visit and hang out with him. It was very important for Mark to keep up with his buddies. His social life was limited, but he grabbed every available second.

Morning after morning, Mark and his parents would leave for Chicago for blood tests and doctor appointments, a round-trip of about 80 miles. On a good day, it might take them an hour and a half each way. Many days, because of traffic, it would be a two- to three-hour commute, a stressful commute for anyone, but especially for Sue and Ray, with Mark in the backseat, bundled up in a blanket, weak and often nauseous. They were all unsure of what each day would bring. The routine of doctor and hospital visits became their new reality.

On one of their many trips to the city, Sue jokingly said to Mark, "If only we had a dime for every trip we made up here. We would be millionaires." This conversation would come up many times over the six years of Mark's treatments.

Before long, Mark was admitted to the hospital for five straight days of chemotherapy. He slept a good deal of the time, and simply walking down the corridor left him winded and fatigued.

Following his discharge, the protocol was every three weeks he would have another round of chemo, and this would continue until five rounds were administered. The week following each treatment, he would always get a fever and need to be re-admitted for antibiotics. Then he would have one week of feeling "normal" until the brutal cycle started all over again.

After several months of treatments, Mark had scans and more tests to determine the progress of his chemotherapy. The doctor asked for a meeting with Sue and Ray. Anxious and nervous, they met with him in the hospital cafeteria.

Mark's oncologist said, "Mark is not responding to treatment as we had hoped and expected." He continued, "We feel we have done all we can for him."

Ray turned to him and asked, "So if nothing more is done how long does he have?"

"Six months."

Sue stood up without speaking; she immediately turned around and walked out. She needed to find a private place. She walked around until she found a small but empty room: a place where she could scream at the top of her lungs; a place where she could cry and not be seen or heard; a place she did not want to go.

Sue and Ray talked; neither was willing to accept the devastating and discouraging prognosis.

They immediately asked for Mark's release and records. Although they did not have a plan, they packed him up and took him home. They knew they would not sit idly by because each of them was filled with determination and hope. These results may have kicked them and knocked them down, but they wouldn't stay down for long.

They were determined to find another doctor, another hospital, where they could find hope. Sue called her brother Kent and told him the news. He immediately began doing research and found a doctor at Children's Memorial Hospital whose specialty was Neuroblastoma. Kent made a few calls, and the hospital agreed to see Mark right away. Within a few days, they admitted him to Children's Memorial Hospital (now Lurie Children's) in Chicago.

For Sue and Ray, a feeling of hope and control returned. They were determined to provide the best medical care for their boy. They understood the move would not be easy but knew they had to push forward to give Mark a fair chance.

Mark was not happy about changing hospitals. The abrupt move confused and terrified him. He had grown close to the nursing staff at his previous hospital and liked his doctors. Moving him was a huge decision and one that Mark resented. They did not think it would help Mark in any way to tell him the details of the meeting. They just told him they'd heard great things about this hospital, and the doctors there were experts in treating kids.

But Mark's attitude shifted. His willingness to cooperate changed, and he dished his anger out to everyone. He argued and refused to eat. He became quiet and withdrawn. It's possible he was in one of those stages in which people become angry and lash out. Fair enough...his world felt totally out of control, and his anger was justified. Although Mark was grumpy and mad at everyone, Sue felt he was more like himself and thought the fight in him was needed to endure the next phase of his journey. She understood Mark would come to terms with the move in his own time.

The move was difficult. Mark was not familiar with the hospital, and this added to his anxiety. In the previous hospital, he'd had a private room, and suddenly he had to share a room with another kid who had cancer. The lack of privacy was an adjustment and hard on all of them.

At his November admission to Children's Memorial Hospital, Mark weighed barely 50 pounds. The doctors determined no further treatment could begin until Mark became stronger and gained weight. He was weak and frightened, and he had no appetite.

Thanksgiving, 2000, was the first holiday Mark would spend in the hospital. A large group of family gathered to spend Thanksgiving with him, and they shared a meal together in the cafeteria. Mark observed it sure wasn't like Mom's cooking, and everyone had a good laugh.

At Children's, the first thing Mark needed was a central line (an IV inserted under general anesthetic for the comfort and convenience of dispensing all medications). Because Mark did not have a central line, each time he needed a test or treatment, medical staff would have to put in an intravenous line. And more than anything, Mark hated being "stuck."

They explained this to Mark as a necessary surgical procedure that would allow him the comfort of not being "stuck" anymore. He was all for it. Mark made them aware of his bad experience with anesthesia, and they assured them they had the best sleepy juice around! The procedure went well, and he was thrilled not to be stuck every time a nurse came into his room.

Mark began a strict nutritional diet and TPN. TPN stands for total parenteral nutrition. It is for patients who cannot get their nutrition through diet alone and is administered through the central line. This procedure provided high calories and protein to boost his weight and strength. Within weeks Mark's weight increased to seventy pounds, and the discussion began for Mark to have his first stem cell transplant, a procedure used to replace damaged or diseased stem cells with healthy cells.

The weight gain was crucial for Mark's treatments to progress. He began to feel stronger, but his lousy attitude remained the same.

CHAPTER NINE: FROM GRUMPY TO GRATEFUL

*"Dear God, please help me not to have
stomach pain anymore. Please help me
to be strong and not to be kranky. Help
me to take my medicines like I should.
Please help me to stay fever free. Please
help my white count go up. Please help
me to be strong enough to do the things
with my family. And please watch over
me and my family and friends. Thank
You for Your many blessings. Amen."*

Mark Staehely

No matter how Mark was feeling, he
continued to write his prayers in a journal and
always expressed his gratitude for his many
blessings. But as Mark's treatment continued, he
became more agitated and difficult for his care
team to treat. Unlike the previous hospital where
the nurses wanted to be assigned to Mark on their
shift, the new staff would rotate each shift so Mark
would have a different nurse each day. They had to
struggle with Mark to take his medication.

On one particular day, Mark once again
refused to take his medication. No amount of
bribing or begging would work. A hospital
volunteer happened to be walking by, and one of
the nurses pulled him aside and asked him to visit
Mark. His name was Don. Don's volunteer work
consisted of getting to know the kids on the
oncology floor. He would spend time chatting,
joking, and developing a relationship with them.
He had a warm smile and a relaxed demeanor.

Don, sixty-six, had been a volunteer at
Children's Memorial Hospital for nine years. He
entered Mark's room and saw a young boy across

the room, glaring at him. Don introduced himself and began to make small talk. Mark gave him one-word answers and refused to engage in the conversation. Don moved closer to the bed and decided he would gamble that Mark liked baseball. Even that topic could not get Mark to respond. Then Don mentioned he was originally from New York and was a huge Boston Red Sox fan.

Suddenly, he saw a glimmer of interest in Mark's eyes. He continued to talk about the team and soon discovered that Mark was also a huge Red Sox fan. In this conversation, Don discovered common ground. An hour quickly passed. Don had other kids to visit but left with a promise to Mark he would be back the next day.

Soon, Mark began looking forward to Don's visits. He would take the medications without fighting. Don and Mark developed a special bond, and with Don's help, Mark began to get his old spark back. This was the beginning of a beautiful friendship. For Don, Mark would do anything.

Mark stopped fighting the nurses, and because of Don and his friendship, he soon began charming everyone again. The nurses began fighting over who would be his nurse for the day!

Chapter Ten: No School

*"Dear God, Please help me not to get a
fever while I'm home. Please help my
counts not to go to low. Please help me
eat and drink. Finally please make me
better really fast. I love You, God.
Amen."*

Mark Staehely

Fall 2000

Each morning I would wake up and open
my shade. I would look out my window and
immediately see the Staehely's house and start my
day with a prayer for their safe travels. On many
mornings, I would see Ray or Michael carry Mark
to the car. They would wrap him in a blanket and
gently buckle him in the back seat. Mark weighed
barely 70 pounds, but Ray's shoulders sagged as he
walked, and Mark looked heavy in his arms. On
those mornings, my heart ached for them.

It would be impossible for me as a parent to
pretend I understood any of this. I was scared on
their behalf, felt useless, and had no idea how to
help. I have a deep belief in the power of prayer,
and as I stood on the outside of their world, I
would pray. Many prayer groups around the
neighborhood and community kept Mark and his
family covered in prayer.

One thing I did understand, though, was
that my fears and worries were nothing compared
to theirs. I would never pretend to comprehend
their journey, yet every day I would look on with
concern and continue to search for hope in my
faith.

Mark spent most of the summer in the
hospital. He would go home for a few days only to

return because they could not stabilize his blood counts. His counts would become a significant struggle, both blood and platelets. He needed transfusions weekly so that he would be strong enough to continue further treatments. Maintaining blood counts became a constant battle for him.

His best friend, JP, was beginning seventh grade, and our son Alex, a year younger, was starting sixth grade. JP and Alex spent a lot of time with Mark during the summer. Once in a while, they were invited to go with Mark to the hospital to keep him company during a transfusion. These day trips continued after school started in the fall, and they would take turns going to the hospital with Mark. The teachers and administrators were very understanding and supportive, allowing JP and Alex to miss classes. Having a buddy along helped make the trip a little easier to tolerate for both Mark and Sue.

Word traveled fast that Mark would not be returning to classes in the fall. Because of his weak immune system, he spent his entire seventh grade school year in and out of the hospital. The kids began sending get well cards home for Mark, through JP or Alex, and this helped him stay connected to his friends. As parents, we talked openly with Alex and JP about Mark's cancer, and we assured them everything was being done to make Mark well. The boys were old enough to understand how serious it was but seemed to dwell more on how they could spend time with him, wanting to make his life as normal as possible by playing video games, watching baseball, and talking.

I would often walk over with Alex to deliver the cards, and Mark would be tucked under blankets on the couch in the family room. I would notice he perked up and sat a little straighter when we visited. During these visits, my relationship with Mark began to grow. He always asked how I was and how Dave and Adam were. He seemed genuinely interested, and I found myself talking to him like a friend about work and sharing funny stories with him.

Mark had a way of making you feel at ease with his illness because he spoke openly about the treatments and about how lousy they were. He never pretended not to be sick, but he mostly wanted to talk about sports or about what was happening at school with Alex and JP. It was obvious to visitors Mark felt nauseous and weak, but he wasn't going to waste a visit dwelling on that. He had his priorities.

The school district assigned a tutor and made every effort to help him to keep up with his school work. On most days, Mark didn't have the energy to listen to, much less concentrate on, a math lesson. After a couple of months, it became apparent Mark could not keep up with the curriculum. The treatments were taking a toll on his energy and strength. Unable to focus, Mark's parents and the school counselors decided to discontinue tutoring so that Mark could get stronger.

Sue and Ray considered buying a computer so that Mark could entertain himself and stay connected to his friends. In 2000, home computers were becoming more common; however, they were costly, and not everyone could afford one. One afternoon, I glanced over at their house and saw several large boxes sitting on their front steps. Making this purchase was a big decision and expense, but one that proved well worth the investment.

Mark missed his entire seventh grade school year at Troy Junior High. Missing school for Mark was more about missing the social aspect than the academics. He desperately missed playing sports, having a girlfriend, and getting into mischief.

Mark always wanted to know what was going on at school. He wanted to hear about the girls and was excited when most of the kids started to get email. He could keep up on all the latest school gossip on Myspace. He maintained and built friendships, thanks to social networking. Ray believed the purchase of the computer proved to be a lifeline for Mark.

Friday night dances and basketball games were a big deal in the lives of these kids. JP's mom, Dee, and I shared the struggle of watching our boys attend these events, knowing Mark was at home. We felt strange and unexplainable guilt, and week after week it continued to bother us. However, not once did Mark whine or complain about missing dances or sports events. His acceptance of his limitations was mature beyond his years.

CHAPTER ELEVEN: CHRISTMAS 2000

*"Dear God, Thank you for today, thank
you for all I've been given today. Thank
you for all that you've done for me
today. Thank you for all my doctors
and nurses that have helped me. Help
me to get stronger and healthier. Help
me to gain weight. Please watch over
my family, friends and I tonight and
forever. Thank you for all your
blessings."*

Mark Staehely

Lurie Children's (then Children's Memorial Hospital) makes every effort to discharge a patient, if at all possible, so that they can spend the holiday at home with their family. The Staehelys were looking forward to spending Christmas together at home, and Mark's counts were back to normal. Home Health Care would visit every few days to check Mark's vitals and draw blood to monitor his red and white blood counts. Friends stopped by and kept Mark company, hanging out and playing video games.

Unfortunately, just days after being discharged, Mark began to feel lethargic and developed a fever. Test results showed this to be an infection, and he needed IV antibiotics. He was readmitted to the hospital and would stay through Christmas.

Mark had many visitors during the Christmas holiday. Each visitor had to wear a gown and mask to protect Mark because of his infection and low white blood counts. On Christmas Day, they shared gifts, which managed to keep him busy and entertained.

Although Mark had many visitors to bring him Christmas cheer, he commented on how many kids were alone on Christmas day. Many of them didn't even have one visitor. He said, "It sucks being in the hospital on Christmas!" No one knew this better than Mark. He saw the nurses and volunteers do what they could to bring a little cheer to the kids without company, but he wanted to do something himself. He got up out of bed, put on a gown and a mask, and rolled his IV pole around the floor, smiling that famous smile and wishing every kid he encountered a Merry Christmas!

This situation impacted Mark in a considerable way that would change his life and the life of every child at Children's Memorial Hospital. After all, these kids were not merely other patients; they were his friends.

CHAPTER TWELVE: 100 DAYS

"Dear God, Thank you for everything you have done for me so far. But now this time is really important, so I'm asking if you would really watch over me these next couple of months, watch over me when I'm having my three transplants not to get to sick and have no reactions please God I know you could help me these hard times. And I thank you and love you lord. Thank you for everything I have asked for. Amen."

Mark Staehely,March 14, 2001 (the only prayer that was dated)

Mark was facing a stem-cell transplant. His stem cells would be harvested and re-implanted. This procedure would take place over several weeks.

There would be three stem-cell transplant procedures; the first two were outpatient, and the third one would be inpatient. For this third transplant, they had to treat Mark with aggressive chemotherapy to kill as many bad cells as possible. This procedure destroyed his white counts but was necessary for his body to receive the transplant. Mark had no appetite and experienced weakness during this time. Due to his compromised immune system, he would be confined in the hospital and at home, in isolation for 100 days.

100 days!

The isolation requirement meant Sue had to sanitize the house entirely for him to return home. Pictures had to be removed from walls, and knick-knacks packed away in boxes. Air vents and carpets had to be professionally cleaned.

The Staehelys lived in a tri-level home with the family room on the lower level. One of the rooms remained unfinished with open insulation and dust. When friends and neighbors heard about this dilemma, they came together. Not only did they fix the problem, but they finished off the level by adding a bedroom, bathroom, and laundry room. They worked frantically to finish the job so that Mark could come home to the cleanest and healthiest environment possible.

No visitors were allowed during this isolation period, except Home Health Care. The "no visitor" rule was tough on the boys, and quite often, when Mark was having a bad day, Sue would bend the rules and let one of the boys come over. JP and Alex were Mark's "go-to" friends. Jonathan, JP's little brother, was also a big part of the friendship mix. He became the little brother Mark never had. If he arrived home from school first, he would often run over and hang out with Mark. If Mark wanted one of them to come over, they would all drop what they were doing and run next door. They each became a reliable lifeline, a distraction from the hospital stays and blood transfusions.

On the days Mark felt well enough, he spent time on the computer. He knew very little about technology but taught himself how to set up email accounts, use Google, and install games. This new hobby became his link to the outside world.

Ray and Mark spent hours online researching baseball and football cards, learning which cards had the highest value and were the rarest to acquire. Because of the internet, a whole new world opened up to Mark, and he taught his dad everything he learned. This hobby became something special for the two of them and proved to be an excellent way to pass the time together.

Ray remembers digging under the seats of the couch and lifting up the car mats, looking for spare change so that he could buy more baseball and football cards. Money remained tight, but when it came to Mark, be it a four-wheeler, a computer, or sports cards, he would find a way. It was that simple.

CHAPTER THIRTEEN: OUR FAMILIES

*"Dear God, I want to thank you for
making the Lindgren family. I believe
Peggy was put on earth for a reason,
that reason is to be a wonderful friend
and person. She is truly an angel. I also
want to thank you for my two best
friends, Adam and Alex. They are truly
amazing friends. And are also angels.
Last but not least, Dave is just
awesome. He was put on earth for a
reason also, so he could be Dad of
Adam and Alex, and the husband of
wonderful Peggy. Thank you for
blessing me with such wonderful
neighbors and friends. Amen."*

Mark Staehely

This particular prayer makes me laugh out loud every time I read it. It touches the very depth of my soul, and I will treasure it always.

During this challenging time of isolation for Mark, my mom passed away. She had been ill for several months, and although we were anticipating her death, we could never really be prepared. We had planned a small memorial service for her at my church. We accepted it was out of the question for Mark to attend the service because of the high risk of infection. However, he had other plans. Remember, he was a stubborn and determined boy. When Mark set his mind to something, it was next to impossible to change it.

Mark insisted he attend the service. Sue said, "Mark, I'm sorry, but you can't go because you are too weak, and being in public could make you sicker." He was only halfway through his isolation period.

She expected this to be the end of the conversation, but he looked her straight in the eye and said, "Either you drive me, or I will start walking."

After the service began, my son Alex tapped my arm, nodding toward the back of the church. I will never forget turning around and seeing Mark, standing there next to his mom, wearing a surgical mask. He waved to me.

I knew what a sacrifice it was for him to be there, and this unselfish act of kindness touched my heart beyond words. He always managed to put others first, even when he physically felt so bad. That was Mark.

Later that day, Mark walked over and handed me this prayer:

> *"Dear God, I need to ask you a few*
> *things to do for me. Could you*
> *please have Peggy's Mom watch*
> *over Peggy, her family and friends.*
> *To help them through the hard*
> *times. Please have her help all of us*
> *to live a great life. Finally, please*
> *help Peggy's Mom to get everything*
> *she wants up there in heaven. Thank*
> *you for all your blessings. Amen"*

Summer 2001

The next summer, Ray bought enough fireworks to put on a first-rate Fourth of July show. He invited our family over to the firework production. We brought over our chairs, snacks, and drinks and anticipated the darkness so Ray could begin the display. Soon, it began, and all you could hear were the "oohs and ahhs."

Ray was really into the action. Suddenly, one of the Roman candles went haywire and shot directly at Mark, who was sitting in a chair with Sue. Everyone scattered and jumped up, falling over each other in the process!

Mark shouted, "Gee Dad, what are you trying to do? Kill me?" Laughter erupted and filled the quiet night with sounds of fun and festivity. Only Mark could turn a near-disastrous situation into one of the funniest memories of all times.

It was during this time that I believe Mark invited our family into his world. That world consisted of great heartache and worries, but somehow Mark managed to move us past that. He was very ill; we all knew that, but Mark embraced life in a way that went beyond our understanding. He was making his life count—one small act of kindness at a time.

Michael and our son Adam were two years apart. They had been friends over the years, and both played baseball. Mike had graduated from high school only two weeks before Mark's diagnosis and was planning to leave for ISU in the fall. However, Mike began having second thoughts and could not imagine being away from Mark. He decided to stay home and attend the local community college. Mike felt it was important to be home, close to Mark and the family, and never regretted his decision.

A year had passed since Mark's diagnosis. It had been a year filled with tests, treatments, and many tribulations. Mark remained the one who held us all up. He was the one who kept us laughing and hoping. Because of him, we all began to understand that Mark was not dying but living life on his terms, with humor, honor, and dignity.

CHAPTER FOURTEEN: MOVING FORWARD

*"Dear God, I will be starting radiation
in a couple of days. I'm asking a few
things. Please help me to be strong and
to go through it really strong. Please
help me to not get sick. Please help me
to be a good boy to my family and
friends. And please bless and Watch
over my family and friends. Thank you
for your blessings. Amen."*

Mark Staehely

Summer turned to fall, 2001, and Mark was anxious to return to school. The stem-cell transplants had taken a huge toll on him; he had little energy and lost all his hair. He lost the weight he had gained before the transplants, and his blood counts were a constant challenge. His scans were not encouraging, but no one, not the doctors nor Mark, was giving up.

After the three stem-cell transplants, Mark began radiation. Dr. John Kalapurakal from Northwestern Memorial Hospital would direct his radiation therapy.

Troy School District continued to stand by Mark, allowing him the flexibility to return to school with his regular class. They accommodated the family in any way possible to support and encourage Mark. He would go to classes on days he felt up to it, and this allowed him to interact with his friends and attend sporting events.

Unfortunately, after only a couple of weeks, it became apparent he was losing strength. His body was not producing enough platelets, and his white count was at an all-time low. This left him at risk for bleeding and other complications. He continued to need frequent blood transfusions and radiation treatments, so once again his days were filled with doctor and hospital visits.

Ray and Mark kept busy and entertained with their baseball and football card collection. They were getting to know the owner of the local store where they bought their cards and discovered he was a volunteer firefighter at Troy Fire Department. Mark told him he dreamed of being a firefighter one day, and they spent a great deal of time talking about the job. Mark loved to hear his stories, and one day a firetruck pulled up to the Staehely house; two firefighters knocked on their door. They invited Mark down to the fire station, where he met the entire crew and got a private tour. This was a dream come true for Mark.

From that day on, he spent as many hours as physically possible getting to know the guys and doing little jobs for them. Mark quickly learned the routine and grasped the deep understanding of the station's brotherhood. The Troy Fire Department made Mark an honorary cadet.

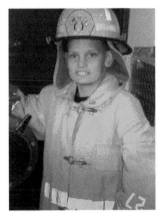

He insisted that Ray buy him a scanner so that he could listen at home for the emergency calls and know what the guys were doing when he wasn't there. Mark would show up after a call and help them wipe down the trucks, asking question after question about the rescue. Being a part of this team gave Mark a new sense of belonging, and he was moving forward.

Chapter Fifteen: The Toy Drive

"If you Give in life it comes back one hundred times over."

Mark Staehely

During the first year of his illness, Mark spent every major holiday in the hospital, except the Fourth of July. On Thanksgiving Day, a large group of family members had gathered in the hospital cafeteria to share a meal. Mark's birthday, December 7th, was another occasion he celebrated in-patient, surrounded by family. Several staff members stopped in to wish him a happy birthday because Mark was well known on the fourth floor. Everyone from the nurses to the staff photographer knew him by name.

Mark often talked about his first Christmas Day in the hospital and how sad it had made him to see so many kids spend the day there. He felt deeply for these kids and would soon make a decision that would change his life and the lives of all who knew him.

December 2001

On a bitterly cold day in the middle of December, our doorbell rang. Mark stood there with a serious look on his face and said he had something to ask me. I quickly invited him in, and he blurted out, "Peggy, I need your help!"

He explained, "I know it's getting close to Christmas, but can we do a toy drive for

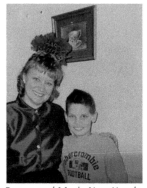

Peggy and Mark, New Year's Eve, 2002

the kids on 4 West?" The fourth floor, the oncology floor, had become his second home.

Mark often talked about his first Christmas in the hospital. He said no matter how many visitors he had; he couldn't stop thinking about all those kids spending the holidays there alone. He described it as "lousy." The nurses do everything they can to make it a special day for the kids, but it is not the same.

He knew his mom was extremely busy and worried about him. He didn't want to tell her his concerns because he thought it would overwhelm her. He was determined and sincere, and I felt honored he wanted my help. Looking into those big blue eyes, I knew right then that there was no answer other than "YES!" We walked right over to his house because he wanted me to be the one to tell his mom.

As soon as we walked in, Sue took in our mischievous expressions. Mark, smiling ear to ear, immediately blurted out his idea, and I quickly assured her I would take care of everything. Of course, standing there with Mark and seeing the hope and enthusiasm on his face melted her heart. She was all for it!

The challenge of bringing Mark's idea to fulfillment became our immediate priority. That night Mark came down with a fever and infection and was urgently admitted to the hospital. He wouldn't be released for five days.

Mark knew I had several close friends at my church that would help carry out his plan. I immediately sent out several emails, and word spread quickly in the neighborhood. The response was amazing: friends and neighbors began dropping off bags and bags of toys! In only a few days, we ended up with over one hundred toys to fill the thirty gift bags needed for the fourth floor. Mark came up with the idea to find out how many kids were inpatients and personalize each bag according to their age and gender.

As soon as Mark was discharged, he walked over to our house and saw the living and dining rooms filled with toys. His eyes grew large, and the smile on his face was priceless. For a split second, he was speechless, but he quickly recovered and shouted "Let's get started!"

That afternoon, with Christmas music

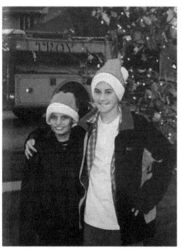

blaring throughout the house, Sue, Mark, Alex, and I sat on the floor of our living room and sorted the toys accordingly. We filled each gift bag with books, games, and toys.

The following week, on Friday, December 21st, we loaded all the gift bags into the back of my van, and off we went to Children's Memorial Hospital. As Mark and Alex donned their Santa hats, they wore the biggest smiles I'd ever seen.

After we arrived on the fourth floor, Mark, a look of pure joy on his face, personally handed a gift bag to each child and wished each and every one a Merry Christmas. He asked for nothing in return but a hug. Forever etched in my mind are the bright smiles on the faces of those children and the laughter that wafted through the halls. No matter how many years have passed, this was the most meaningful Christmas of my life and a favorite holiday memory. For me and many others, Mark was the true spirit of Christmas, and for a few minutes, his illness was forgotten and joy filled our hearts.

Sue, Mark, Alex, and Peggy, 2001

Our local paper, the *Joliet Herald News*, heard about this young boy with cancer doing a toy drive for his friends in the hospital. They came out with a photographer and interviewed us for the article. This would be one of many articles in the years that followed finding Mark a newsworthy topic.

We had no idea that this would be the beginning of the famous Mark Staehely Toy Drive.

CHAPTER SIXTEEN: MARK, THE TEACHER

*"No matter what happens in life, don't
ever give up. Keep trying."*

Mark Staehely

Mark not only changed the lives of hundreds of children through his unselfish acts of kindness but also touched the hearts of many adults.

In January, 2002, following the article in the *Joliet Herald News*, Mark received a letter from Mr. Larry Wiers, Troy School District Superintendent. The letter expressed his pride and admiration for Mark. Mark treasured this letter and felt honored that someone like Mr. Wiers had taken notice of him! Mr. Wiers assisted the family in Mark's transition back to Troy Middle School.

Mr. Wiers sat down with Sue and Ray in the Summer of 2002. They discussed what would be in Mark's best interest moving forward in the school year. It was decided that Mark would continue eighth grade. JP was moving on to high school. It was fortunate for Mark to be in classes with Alex.

In the fall of 2002, Mark returned to school and the eighth grade. On the first day, the marquee greeted him with "Welcome Back, Mark." Mr. Wiers met Mark at the front door and let him know that anytime he was having a bad day, he was welcome to go down to his office and chat. During these many conversations, they became close friends. Mark would attend classes when he felt up to it, and the entire student body welcomed Mark back with open arms.

I had the opportunity to visit with Mr. Wiers and listen to his many insights about Mark.

Mr. Wiers retired from Troy School District in 2007. He is an adjunct professor in the College of Education at Lewis University in Romeoville, Illinois. Mr. Wiers has dedicated his life to the betterment of education and continues to inspire future teachers. He believes education is the greatest profession in the world as it continues to enrich a person for his or her whole life. He has lectured and spoken to hundreds of students over the years, and Mark has been his inspiration and the topic of many of these lectures.

"Why Mark?" I asked Larry. He explained that he'd taught for many years before becoming an administrator and knew thousands of kids over the years. What made Mark different? Mark immediately impressed him with how 'other-centered' he was. He understood the mindset of this age group and the natural way they focused on their own being. Kids this age are typically learning to get better at being themselves and are self-centered and growing into their personalities. But he found in Mark's case it was totally the opposite. He said, "Teaching is about the service industry." What struck him about Mark was that he was already in the "service" industry at such a young age. His toy drive was evidence of this.

He commented, "Mark did more for others in his illness than many of us do in good health."

Something else about Mark struck Mr. Wiers: they were both sports fans. Larry especially loves the Chicago White Sox. He and Mark had that in common. They spent a great deal of time talking sports, and Mark knew statistics, which both impressed and intrigued Mr. Wiers.

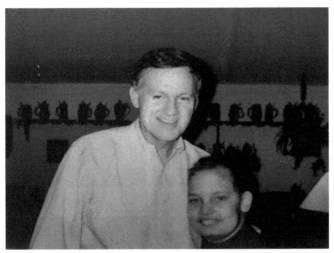

Mr. Wiers at Mark's 16th birthday party

Quite often, Mr. Wiers would attend one of the many sporting events for the Middle School. One day, he sat next to Mark in the stands at a baseball game. He understood Mark loved to play the game and knew he was an All-Star player; in an ideal world, Mark would have been out on that field, playing the game he loved. Larry was impressed that Mark sat there cheering for his buddies and witnessed him demonstrating his "other-centeredness."

As he sat in the bleachers with Mark, he said, "You know, Mark, I give a lot of talks to students and adults. And in my talks, I speak about the quality of perseverance, how it's the greatest gift a human being can have because we are all guaranteed to face failure in our lives."

He continued, "It's the people who react and respond to setbacks the quickest that are the most successful." He mentioned how he saw that great quality of perseverance in Mark. He said, "I have to tell you that one of the people in my talks is Abraham Lincoln, who faced nothing but adversity yet rose to the highest office in the land. I also speak about Colonel Harland Sanders, who at age 65 still hadn't discovered his recipe after 1008 attempts only to have his recipe accepted on his 1009th try!" Mr. Wiers told Mark about a few other famous people he referenced, and then he turned to Mark and said, "Mark, you will be in my talk."

Mark responded, "Aww, no..."

Mr. Wiers said, "Yes, Mark, you will be in that talk. I'm going to talk about you as an example of perseverance." He described the pictures of all these people that he showed on a big screen behind him. "I need your picture, and I need your advice."

As luck would have it that day, the school photographer was there taking pictures of the baseball team in action for the yearbook. Mr. Wiers called her over and told her he needed a picture of Mark. Then he turned to Mark and asked, "What advice would you give everybody I talk to about perseverance?" Then Mark gave him his advice.

"No matter what happens in life, don't ever give up. Keep trying! Try to help as many people as you can because I believe it will help you reach your goals in life."

Larry looked at me and said, "Peggy, no way an eighth grader with Neuroblastoma, facing this kind of adversity, would ever give a quote like this."

As we sat there, tears filled our eyes; we both understood the power behind those words, out of the mouth of a young boy who had an old soul. We realized this is not a typical quote from someone so young; it was exceptional. Larry recognized this as one of those "God moments" his pastor spoke of so often.

Larry had a bookmark made with the picture of Mark taken that day at the ballfield printed on the front. Mark's quotes surround the picture, and on the back are these words from Mr. Wiers:

"Every morning for the past 52 years I have gotten up and gone to school. In that time, I don't know if I have seen or had a better teacher than Mark. Mark has taught us lessons you cannot find in a textbook. In an 'up close and personal' way, Mark has taught us courage, love, service, and persistence. He has stared down adversity and pain and showed us how to minister to others in need. Mark did more, served more, loved more in his illness than most do in good health. He was the personification of persistence. He will forever be an inspiration to all of us touched by his incredible life."

Larry Wiers
September 9, 2006

Larry distributed hundreds of these bookmarks over the years.

In 2005, Larry Wiers nominated Mark for the American Red Cross Youth Good Samaritan Award, Youth Good Samaritan Category. He believed Mark's outstanding Good Samaritan work and extraordinary heroism should be recognized. He won! The award was for youth under the age of twenty-one who acted selflessly when helping another in need, performed an act of heroism involving an unusual, significant, or unexpected incident that required a courageous reaction in a crisis, or made an ongoing commitment to the community through acts of kindness, courage, or unselfishness.

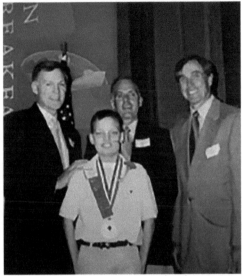

Mark accepting the Hometown Hero award with Larry Wiers (left) Ray, Mark's dad (center), and Dick Jauron (right)

Mark was presented this award at the Third Annual Hometown Heroes Breakfast, June 22, 2005, in Chicago, with his family and Mr. Wiers as his guest. The presentation ceremony marked one of the greatest days of their lives.

The ceremony was held at the Hyatt Regency in Chicago. Mark met Mr. Wiers at the door.

"Come on," Mark said. "I want to introduce you to somebody. You are going to be sitting at our table with him." Larry agreed and followed Mark. "Mr. Wiers," Mark said casually, "I would like you to meet Dick Jauron."

A huge Chicago Bears fan, Larry Wiers felt like a kid. Having breakfast with Dick Jauron was a moment he would always remember. Mark receiving the American Red Cross Hometown

Hero award would be one of the proudest moments in both of their lives.

Mark mixed with anyone and everyone, whether it be Dick Jauron, Sammy Sosa, or Nomar Garciaparra, both players for the Chicago Cubs. He could talk to strangers in the grocery store, a homeless person standing on the corner, or a news reporter. Mark, smiling, chatty, and at ease talking with anyone, would draw you into his world.

I asked Mr. Wiers how Mark graduated without completing the necessary academic requirements. He explained that decision by outlining his theory of a teacher's responsibility. During his many talks with new teachers, he told them there are two things not in the job description he expected out of them:

#1) He expects them to be the great revealer. When asked what that meant he explained, "Our work as teachers is to reveal the goodness and greatness in every child. There is a success story in each child waiting to be revealed and told."

#2) It's about giving hope. "We should dispense hope, create possibilities for kids, so they know they are worthy of something greater."

He said, "Quite honestly, an educator considers the whole child, and the whole child is more than just the academic child." Larry had met thousands of kids through the years, but none were like Mark. Especially in Mark's situation, there was so much more to him than the books.

Mr. Wiers told me that if he had not been so moved and inspired by Mark, he would not have been able to talk with me. He embraced every opportunity to talk about Mark.

Finally, I asked Larry to use one word to describe Mark; he thoughtfully answered, "A treasure."

Our interview ended with a hug and with our hearts full of inspiration.

CHAPTER SEVENTEEN: BRUSH WITH FAME

*"Dear God, Please help me stay fever
free. Please help my body fight off all
germs. Please help me to stay strong so
I can spend time with my family and
friends. Please help me to help as many
people as I can. Also please help me to
take all my medicine like I should
everyday. And finally please help me to
get a good night sleep. Thank you God
for all my blessings. Amen."*

Mark Staehely

After his first toy drive, Mark gained a great deal of attention. His outreach to each child did not surprise those closest to Mark or the staff at the hospital. Everyone witnessed his many unselfish acts of kindness over the months during his hospital stays.

Kathleen Keenan, Director of Communications and Media Strategist at Children's Memorial Hospital, stated in an interview, "He is truly teaching us that at any age you can turn a negative into positive and bring the spirit of Christmas to life...He has overcome amazing challenges. He teaches us all what Christmas is all about. At any age, you can not only make a difference, but you can also move hearts and souls."

Mark drew attention from sports figures, who were also his personal heroes, from the media that flourished on this kind of heart-warming story, and from authority figures who thrived on the positive impact this young boy had on so many people.

Sports Figures

Chicago Bears

Famous sports figures often visit children who are patients in large hospitals. These visits are excellent public relations, but the difference they make to a child is remarkable. This was the case when Chicago Bears Head Coach, Dick Jauron, who coached the Bears for five seasons (1999-2003), and his wife visited Mark. One day while making their usual rounds, they entered Mark's room. There was no need for an introduction as Mark knew Coach Jauron immediately and perked right up. He had plenty of advice for the coach and made a lasting impression. Mark told Coach Jauron that the offensive line needed some work and gave him specific instructions.

A few days later, following another tough football loss, Sue woke up to five huge, muscular men standing in Mark's room. Sue woke Mark up, and he recognized them as Bears offensive linemen. They introduced themselves anyway and told Mark that Coach Jauron had sent them for any and all tips Mark could offer. Without hesitation, Mark shared his thoughts. Sue remembered the excitement and confidence in his voice as he told each of them what they must do and the changes that should occur.

Coach Jauron made it possible for Mark and a few of his friends to attend the Bears Training Camp in Bourbonnais. The boys were given first-class attention, including a special golf cart. After lunch with the players, they spent time with Brian Urlacher. They treasured that day and had plenty of autographs and sports memorabilia to show for it. Over the years, long after Coach Jauron left Chicago, he stayed in close touch with the Staehely family.

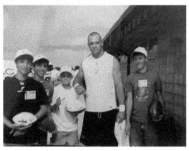

Brian Urlacher with Mark and friends

Chicago White Sox

Christine O'Reilly, Vice President of Community Relations for the Chicago White Sox and Executive Director of Chicago White Sox Charities, often visited children at the hospital. Introducing Christine to Mark was Tom Sullivan, President of the Children's Memorial Hospital Foundation (now known as Lurie Children's Foundation).

As they entered Mark's room, Sue remembers Mark sitting up a little bit taller. After the introductions, Mark looked directly into Christine's sparkling blue eyes and said, "Wow, you are beautiful!"

She replied, "Thank you, Mark. I hear you are a huge White Sox fan." Christine suggested Mark might enjoy attending a game. She soon became one of Mark's closest friends.

At the park, White Sox players made Mark feel extra special, Carl Everett being one of these guys. Carl shared his private number with Mark, and they had several conversations. Carl always took the time to visit with Mark and encourage him.

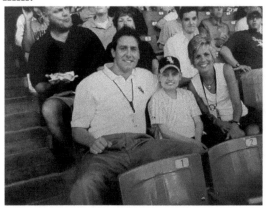

One day Christine was visiting Mark, and they were once again talking baseball. In 2004, the Boston Red Sox had won

Ryan Gribble, Mark, and Christine at a White Sox game

the World Series. Mark told Christine that he had always been a Boston Red Sox fan, so she made it possible for the family to attend a game between the White Sox and the Red Sox. It was early in the 2005 season, and management allowed Mark to go down on the field so that he could hang out in the dugout with the team. But Mark kept glancing over at the Boston Red Sox dugout.

Christine, reading Mark's mind, explained to him, "Mark, we never, ever approach the opposing team. EVER!" She told him they could observe their batting practice from a distance but could not visit the players.

Before she knew it, David Ortiz, known as Big Papi, walked over to Mark. Jason Varitek and half the team came over, shaking hands and chatting with him. Mark, laughing and smiling, told them how great they were. Christine just stood there, speechless! She laughed and said, "It was the craziest thing! Like he was the Pied Piper."

She found it fascinating that others were drawn to Mark the same way she had been.

In 2005, Mark attended several White Sox games, thanks to Christine. They had an incredible winning season and made it into the World Series. Mark and his family went to the first World Series game at US Cellular Field to watch his beloved White Sox play. Mark was so weak he had to be carried to the stadium in a blanket. Ray remembers picking Mark up so he could cheer with the crowd. That was a very good day, but sadly, once again hospitalized for an infection, he had to watch them win the World Series from his hospital room.

During a news conference following the White Sox World Series victory parade in 2005, Ozzie Guillen mentioned he had to visit a sick kid in the hospital. The sick kid turned out to be Mark. No doubt, he wanted to share a part of the victory with Mark.

Chicago Cubs

Mark's all-time favorite baseball player was Nomar Garciaparra. He played most of his career for Mark's favorite baseball team, the Boston Red Sox. When the Red Sox traded him to the Cubs on July 31, 2004, Mark was excited to have him close by and hoped for an opportunity to see him play.

Children's Memorial Hospital Foundation President Tom Sullivan knew what a big baseball fan Mark was. He stopped by to see Mark in Day Hospital (a program that provides treatment during the day and allows the patient to return home at night) with tickets to a Cubs game that night. Mark was finishing getting platelets and would be able to attend the game if they left immediately following the procedure. With four tickets in hand, Mark and Sue invited his buddy Don, who was a huge Cubs fan and one of his nurses, to join him.

Mark and his guests received VIP treatment. This included great seats and a visit to the Cubs' dugout before the game to watch batting practice. Several players took the time to walk over to Mark and introduce themselves. Mark, wide-eyed and engaged in conversation, proudly wore his favorite Garciaparra jersey. He hadn't noticed that Nomar was absent.

Sue realized it was only a matter of time before Mark began to search for Nomar. She observed Jim Hendry, the General Manager, speaking to the team. She seized the opportunity to introduce herself and asked if Nomar would be coming down for batting practice. Mr. Hendry explained that Nomar had taken early batting practice and would not be down until game time. Sue casually mentioned that Nomar was Mark's all-time favorite player, and he had hoped to meet him. She wished Hendry good luck on the game and went to join Mark.

A few minutes later, Sue saw Nomar walk down the steps into the dugout. With Mark's back to him, he mouthed *shh* to Sue and quietly slid up on the bench next to him. Mark sensed someone sitting close to him and turned his head. His eyes grew large, and that smile broke through.

He asked, "Nomar, is that really you?"

Nomar laughed and said, "Yes, it really is me." He borrowed a pen from Sue and signed the back of Mark's jersey. Then he asked Sue for a piece of paper and wrote down his name and cell phone number for Mark. He told him, "You call me whenever you want to."

Sue chuckled and said, "Oh boy, you may regret that!"

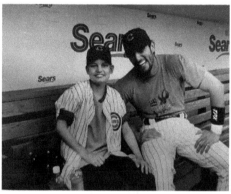

Mark with Nomar Garciaparra

The following week, Mark wanted to call Nomar, and Sue told him, "Mark, he's a busy man."

Mark reminded her, "He said I could call him whenever I want to." Nomar answered on the first ring, and they spoke for a few minutes, Mark wishing him luck on his game. Mark even called him on New Year's Eve, ignoring Sue's hesitation and once again reminding her, "Mom, I can call him anytime."

Kerry Wood was another player who took a special interest in Mark. He was Mark's favorite pitcher, and meeting him was another dream come true. Mark had followed Kerry's career from his beginning with the New York Yankees to the Cleveland Indians and, finally, his fourteen years with the Chicago Cubs. Kerry was wonderful to Mark and made an effort to stay in touch with him.

Media and People in High Places

Mark often acted as an ambassador for the hospital and became acquainted with Chicago Mayor Richard M. Daley. Then, in 2004, WGN radio's Steve Cochran named Mark his "Kid of the Week." Also in 2004, WLS-TV's Harry Porterfield proclaimed Mark to be "Someone You Should Know."

In 2005, Mark was honored for his toy drive by the Children's Memorial Hospital's Board of Directors with their highest award, the George D. Kennedy Distinguished Leadership Award. That year, Mark's toy drive became the largest individual event of its kind without any corporate sponsorship to benefit Children's Memorial Hospital.

At the award ceremony, Mark approached the stage in a wheelchair and with an NG tube (a nasogastric tube, inserted for feeding) and accepted his award from CEO Patrick Magoon. Mark told the audience of CEOs, board members, and hospital supporters, "I'm not doing anything special; I'm just doing what everyone else should be doing." He received a standing ovation.

All the major networks reported on Mark's toy drive. Frank Mathie from Chicago's ABC Channel 7 News was consistent in his reporting of Mark's toy drive, year after year. He often told Sue it was his favorite story of the year.

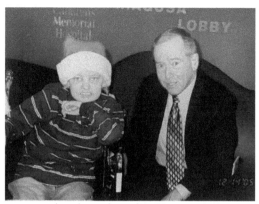

Mark with Frank Mathie, 2005 Toy Drive

For five years Mark participated in the Eric and Kathy Radiothon. This radiothon on 101.9 FM, The Mix, raised money for Children's Memorial Hospital. Year after year, Mark and his family would get up early and drive to Chicago for the radiothon. He loved being in the spotlight, regardless of how miserable he was feeling. One year he did a special shout out to all firemen, and the phones started ringing off the hook. Mark would plead with listeners, and the response was always overwhelming.

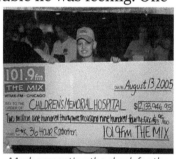

Mark presenting the check for the 2005 radiothon

A special memory for Sue and Ray was during the last radiothon Mark was a guest on the show. He reached in his back pocket and pulled out a wad of money. They had no idea what Mark was about to do. He handed it over to Eric and said, "Here, this is from me."

Sue was shocked. She said, "Mark, you've been saving that money for a while; I thought you had something in mind you wanted to buy for yourself."

Mark quickly responded, "Nope, this is what I want to do."

Sue and Ray will be forever grateful for the many celebrities and personalities who took the time to get to know Mark. He managed to wiggle his way into the hearts of these people unintentionally, yet captured their attention and friendships. Mark accepted every opportunity to be in the spotlight. On good days and bad, he delighted in his brush with fame as long as it put a smile on someone's face.

CHAPTER EIGHTEEN: FRIENDS

"Dear God, I want to thank you for my friends. Thank you for my friends who help me when I'm sad or down or when I am feeling sick. Thank you for my friends, because I have someone to talk to and trust, friends that you can tell secrets to. Friends that you can cry with, friends that stick up for you when your getting made fun of. Thanks for my friends and will you please watch over them. Thank you for all your blessings. Amen."

Mark Staehely

Friends became Mark's lifeline to a world beyond cancer. More than anything, he enjoyed spending time with them. When I began writing this book, I knew there were several people that I needed to speak with, interview, and share their stories.

In reality, everyone who knew Mark had a story to tell. I decided to talk to Sue, and she helped me narrow it down. Friends of Mark had no age, race, or gender base. He could find common ground with anyone and build that into a lasting friendship.

Christine

Christine O'Reilly became one of Mark's closest friends after meeting him when he was a patient at the hospital.

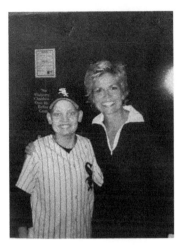

Mark and Christine

Christine was someone who influenced the quality of Mark's life, and she was willing to share her memories and stories with me. She remembered a brightness and lightness about Mark and immediately wanted to get to know him. She felt drawn to him in a way she had not experienced before with any other patient.

She found herself compelled to spend more time with Mark. After her second visit, she rose to leave, and he said, "I love you."

She replied, "I love you too, Mark." He told her you only have to meet someone twice to know you love them.

On days when Mark felt strong enough, Christine would make it possible for Mark to attend a Chicago White Sox baseball game. The time he spent on the field with the players during batting practice was the happiest she ever experienced with him.

She said, "It was the strangest thing: quite often I explained to the players there was a visiting patient, and suddenly without any prodding or explanation, the players walked over to Mark and began talking." This had never happened with previous visitors. She continued, "People were drawn to Mark like I have never seen before."

Meeting Mark was a profound and personal experience. Christine smiled and said, "He had me at hello, and I 'fell in love' with him. He had an illumination about him and didn't even have to try to draw you in. It was like serendipity, a connection to him that was peace and love."

Christine told me she is not overly religious but felt as if she saw the face of God in Mark. She believes there are people on this earth whom some of us have the blessing to meet. That was her experience with Mark. He left an indelible "Mark" on her life.

During our interview, she suddenly got very quiet and said, "Let's talk about Sue and Ray for a minute. They embraced everyone and were selfless and amazing to share Mark with all of us."

I could hear the love and tenderness in Christine's voice as she spoke about him. She summed it up like this: "You can't talk about Mark without feeling there was a magnitude about him and his freedom to love, live, and serve. It was so easy for him, like breathing in and breathing out. He made all of us who knew him better people, and he was just a kid." She laughed and said, "He was a verb, not a noun.!"

Although she shared only a couple of years with Mark, she impacted him as much as he made a difference to her.

She added, "In those precious two years, he touched me and left a mark on my heart for which I am forever grateful."

Childhood Friends

Mark's closest buddies were Alex (my youngest son), JP, and his younger brother Jonathan. I felt the strength of their friendship, and the impact it made on their adult lives is vital to share. I saw firsthand how these boys interacted with each other and how profound their bonds were. As they grew closer during Mark's illness, their relationships would shape the men they would one day become.

Many days the boys would ride their bikes. Outings such as riding bikes or playing outside where she couldn't see them always concerned Sue. If Mark fell, it could be devastating because of his constant low-platelet count. Mark would beg her to ride bikes with the boys. We learned later the boys would go one street over and ride their bikes down a massive dirt hill. It's a good thing we were not aware of these wild pranks at the time! The boys remembered trying to talk Mark out of it, but he was always the determined leader. Luckily for them all, he never came home with a single scratch.

Mark had a PICC line (a peripherally inserted central catheter), which is for many purposes, such as administering medications and repeated IV blood draws. Once removed, Mark was allowed to swim. He especially loved to be in the pools around the neighborhood. His joy, combined with his daredevil attitude, continued to show us nothing would stop him from having fun, not even cancer.

The boys loved to roughhouse, and as boys often do, things sometimes got carried away and a little intense. The rougher, the better. When one of them would pin Mark down to the ground or was about to win the game, Mark would shout, "Hey, lighten up! I have cancer, remember?" Not only did he get a huge laugh, but he also took advantage of the situation and always won!

JP

JP had been Mark's best friend since they were toddlers and lived across the street from each other. Growing up, they spent hours and hours playing neighborhood sports, collecting baseball cards, and making Sue take them for their favorite food, McDonald's. They also got into plenty of trouble together. The boys were inseparable and "thick as thieves," as JP fondly recalls.

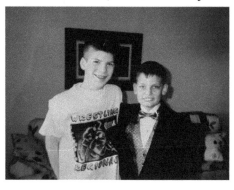

JP and Mark

JP vividly remembers when his mom, Dee, told him and his brother Jonathan to sit down. She explained about Mark's diagnosis. He said there were tears, questions, and concerns instantly. He immediately went over to the Staehely house and saw many of Mark's friends and relatives gathered together. They were hugging and crying. It was intense. He left his best friend's house knowing Mark was in for a fight, and he would be there for him, no matter what.

"JP," I asked, "how do you reflect on your relationship with Mark?" He thoughtfully answered, "I consider myself blessed to have known Mark and to have been his friend. He was the type of friend that always had your back even if he knew you were in the wrong. Mark was a genuine and loving person. He always put others before himself, and he showed it all the time. Mark taught me that no matter how bad a day, week, or even year you are having, someone else was having a worse time than you. Mark also taught me how to be charitable, live life to the fullest every day, and how to be a true friend."

I then asked, "What do you want people to know about Mark?"

JP responded, "The one thing people might not realize about Mark is that he was a true competitor. Everything was a competition to Mark. Whether it was sports, fantasy sports, board games, or even grades in school, Mark wanted to win or beat you. If he couldn't beat you, he was going to put up one hell of a fight."

JP continues, "I believe this was the reason Mark was able to battle this cruel disease for so long. Doctors were always amazed by Mark's progress, but it was the competitor in him that kept him going. I always say Mark didn't let cancer beat him; his body just couldn't take it anymore. Mark was truly one of a kind, and the number of people who knew and loved him showed it. His charismatic and loving personality made it hard not to like Mark."

Alex

Alex and Mark had been childhood friends and grew much closer as teens after Mark's diagnosis. They were able to spend a great deal of time together throughout his illness.

Because of Mark, Alex chose his career as a firefighter/paramedic. He said, "I believe Mark was my biggest inspiration. The passion, persistence, and courage this young man showed through his time with us are unmatched by any other person I have ever met."

Kids ages twelve, eleven, and

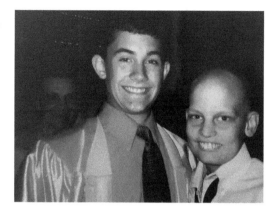

Alex and Mark at Middle School Graduation

eight can't possibly wrap their minds around a friend with cancer. Mark's cancer strengthened their friendships, and Alex felt they came together to help Mark beat his cancer as a team. Each boy did his best to help him any way they could and tried to keep his spirits high so that he could continue to fight.

I asked Alex, "How did Mark influence your life?"

He responded, "Mark influenced my life in many ways. Not only did he show me through his actions how to be more compassionate towards other people in need, but he embodied what it meant to be selfless. There was never any true self-pity although he was known to milk his dad for a few extra bucks for baseball/football cards."

He continued, "I like to believe that I was a good friend to Mark, but I wish I could have told him how much of an impact he truly had on my life. He had a real passion for the fire service, which influenced my career choice; I hope it makes him smile down on me. He believed that helping people in need was paramount, whether at the hospital or in their homes. He taught me nothing is promised in this world and to help one another any way we can along the way.

I learned a lot from Mark, but compassion and perseverance were the greatest lessons. I will always look back on our friendship with happiness and am forever grateful for the time we got to spend together and for the role he played in making me the man I have become today."

Jonathan

Jonathan, four years younger than Mark, became one of Mark's closest friends. As the older boys entered high school, Jonathan and Mark spent many hours together. Age didn't matter, and the influence Mark had on Jonathan was life-changing.

I asked Jonathan about the difference in their ages.

He replied, "JP and Alex were close to Mark in age and school, and I was always the youngest one trying to follow my big brother and his friends around. I became the little brother Mark never had. In my family, and around our neighborhood, there were a lot of boys. Picking on each other was always a way to show one another that you cared about them, as weird as that is. Being the youngest of the whole group, I took my fair share, but again, all out of love. After Mark's diagnosis, that aspect changed greatly. It became a very loving and thoughtful relationship. Mark was always looking out for me. If my brother teased me, Mark would stand up for me."

Johnathan spent hours with Mark in his side room looking at football or baseball cards and just talking. Ray would take them to K's (a local store) to get packs of sport cards to try to find some rare ones for his collection.

He said, "I started spending as much time with him as possible. Sue and Ray would always tell me I was his little buddy."

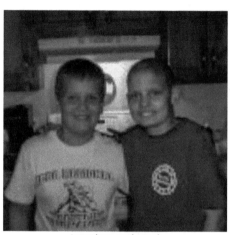
Jonathon and Mark

"Another thing that changed throughout his illness was the almost-celebrity that Mark became. He did all these wonderful things and became a hero to so many people. I was there one day when Nomar Garciaparra called him. That was incredible. He became much more than just a friend or neighbor to me. He became my hero and inspiration."

I asked Jonathan, "What else would you like to share about Mark?"

He replied, "Knowing Mark Staehely and being his friend was one of the greatest blessings in my life. He had the biggest influence on me and who I am today. I still look to him for courage and guidance in times of need. I was only in eighth grade when Mark died, right before high school. A tough age in life, and it broke me. But after watching Mark fight like hell for his life, I knew I could make it through. Because of Mark, no matter what I'm going through, I know I need to persevere, and things will get better. I am forever grateful to him for helping mold me into the man I am today. The feeling you would get from Mark on his good days was indescribable. His personality and positivity were infectious."

In closing, Jonathan added, "It was an honor and a blessing to have had the chance to call Mark not only a friend but a brother. I will never forget him, and thank God I had him in my life, even for a short time. I live out-of-town now, and each time I am home, I try to go to the cemetery and sit and talk to him for a while. There are many times when I can feel Mark's presence, and I know he is there with me. I truly look forward to seeing him again one day."

By now, you know Mark was a unique person. Most teenage boys tend to keep their emotions in check and don't speak or express their love for one another. Mark transformed these friends. He never left a friend without a hug and an "I love you." These words became as natural for these kids as giving each other a high-five. JP, Alex, and Jonathan remember the ease with which Mark expressed his love for them. This expression was a simple yet thoughtful gesture that changed the way they say goodbye to their family and friends still today.

Chapter Nineteen: My Radiation Prayer

"Dear God, I will be starting radiation
in a couple of days. I'm asking a few
things. Please help me to be strong and
go through it really strong. Please help
me to not get sick. Please help me to be
a good boy to my family and friends.
And please bless and Watch over my
family and friends. Thank you for your
blessings. Amen."

Mark Staehely

Mark's treatments consisted of chemotherapy and many medications. Some were new and experimental, but none did anything except make him nauseous and miserable. Nothing could control his pain.

The doctors at Children's Memorial Hospital referred Mark to Dr. John Kalapurakal, Radiologist/Oncologist at Northwestern Memorial Hospital. Dr. John does neuroblastoma research partially supported by the money raised by the Make Your Mark Foundation. They are generous in their funding for this research. He is also the Radiation/Oncology chair for Children's Oncology Group in Chicago. Due to collaborative efforts worldwide, cure rates have gone up for all cancers, including neuroblastoma.

Dr. John, as Mark called him, was more than Mark's doctor. He became a close friend to Mark and the family. He provided personal and professional attention and always did everything in his power to ease Mark's pain. One of the treatments he used was external beam radiation.

According to the American Cancer Society, external beam radiation is used as part of the treatment regimen after a stem cell transplant. Children with high-risk neuroblastoma, like Mark, often need radiation to destroy any cells that remain behind after chemotherapy, as it uses high energy beams to destroy those cells. Radiation can also help relieve pain caused by advanced neuroblastoma.

Mark received high doses of chemotherapy and completed his stem cell transplant. The next step in his protocol entailed five days of radiation therapy.

A few years ago, I was introduced to Dr. John at one of the Make your Mark benefits and decided to reconnect with him for an interview for several reasons. First, it was essential to Sue for me to understand the relationship Mark and Dr. John shared over the years. And as his doctor, Dr. John knew better than anyone what Mark experienced and endured.

For this interview, I prepared a few questions but quickly discovered Dr. John had quite a bit to say about Mark. I just had to listen and learn.

I wondered if Dr. John recalled their first meeting, and he chuckled and replied, "Upon walking in the room, I thought, just another child with cancer, like I have seen hundreds of times before in my practice." At first glance, he saw nothing more than that. He soon discovered Mark would be like no other patient he had ever treated.

As they introduced themselves, it struck him that this patient was different. He said, "Mark was very assertive and very probing of his questions of me. He asked me how long I had been doing this and how good I was." We both laughed at this, remembering how candid Mark could be!

He told Mark, "This is quite unusual; it's like a job interview." He recalled he had to step out right at that moment, and when he returned a few minutes later, Sue said, "Mark already likes you."

"You could not suppress Mark. No inhibitions. He had questions and expected honest answers. He was direct. That first interview was intense, and once I passed Mark's test, I never saw that side of him again. He knew he could die. He wanted to be sure he was coming to a good doctor, and he needed someone who would make his case. He wanted honesty. It began this way, but once he knew who I was, he never questioned me again. But those first few minutes were intimidating, even for this doctor.

"One thing was very clear; Mark was not to be pushed around. He was strong in his character and perhaps far beyond his age." That brief introduction gave Dr. John insight into Mark's strength and level of maturity, and those far exceeded his chronological age. He said, "Mark was a child only in age, and he had a true sense of who he was and was in every other respect one of the kindest adults I had ever met. He was not someone you could push around."

He never had a young patient speak to him that way. Mark was objective in how he spoke, which Dr. John felt was very uncharacteristic of a young patient. He asked Mark, "Am I good enough to treat you?" and Mark answered, "Yes!"

"You see one patient like this in a lifetime, and over thirty years, I have never seen a child like Mark since: none before and none after."

Dr. John spoke of his connection with Mark. "What is most beneficial for a doctor and a patient and the family is for the child and parent to be inquisitive and the doctor willing to listen. It fosters conversation regarding what the hopes, the

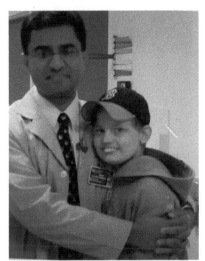
Dr. John and Mark

expectations, the risks, and the benefits are to treat a patient. It's a meaningful discussion and adds value to everyone in the room. The experience intimidates most children, and it is the parents who speak with me. This was not the case with Mark.

"The initial radiation treatment was with curative intent." We discussed how Mark's treatment throughout became constant as the standard protocol did not apply to Mark's case. He would have a couple of good months here and there. "My department was available and on-call for Mark, twenty-four/seven, and we would drop everything for Mark and get him in for treatment within a moment's notice." If Mark told Sue he needed radiation, she would call Dr. John and say, "We are coming," and without hesitation, he would agree.

Mark had more radiation than any other patient Dr. John remembers. He can't count the number of treatments but explained radiation was used for Mark's pain management.

He continued, "That was the kind of relationship we had with him. Why, you wonder, did we have such a special relationship with him? It was not only his magnetic personality, but with Mark, it was because of his generous spirit."

One particular visit, Mark approached Dr. John and shouted, "I see two of you!" Dr. John, fully aware the tumor in Mark's skull caused double vision, replied, "That's my wife's worst nightmare!" They shared a good laugh at Mark's expense, and Dr. John commented on his quick wit. This was the essence of their doctor/patient relationship.

He continued, "We got to know him as a very generous person, always thinking about others and other children, and always more concerned about the other child in the room. Yet he was suffering so much, in so much pain. There have been few adults that have impressed me as being as selfless as Mark. It is very hard to think of somebody else when you are suffering from a terminal condition, and you are in so much pain, and then there was Mark."

Dr. John stopped talking for a minute, and I could tell he was reflecting. Then he said, "For this young kid to have a heart as big as he had when he was suffering and in so much pain, to me is unimaginable. I would never be like that; I could never bear that kind of pain.

"Many adults handle their suffering very well, but I have never seen an adult or child think of others when they are suffering so. Mark always thought and asked about the other patients in the room when he came to see me, like no other patient I have ever had. He never asked me if there was something I could do for him. Not once."

"Most patients are too busy, too focused on their pain. This is normal; this is okay and expected. Nothing is wrong with that for that is how we are as human beings. That's not how Mark was.

"Mark had room in his heart. In spite of his sickness and his illness, in spite of his constant suffering and pain, constant treatment, and therapy, he was always thinking about the other guy. How could he do that? Did that kind of heart ease his suffering? Make him well? What prompted him to be that way? Was that kind of caring or kind thoughts any value to him? Any use? Would it help him live longer? Not that I know. I'm sure it did spiritually; that is why he was so different. How could he fill his life with the kind of grace he offered to others as a young boy? Mark somehow channeled his goodness and grace and did better than most patients with this illness.

"I know for a fact I have never seen anyone like him. Not in my family or my practice.
"I tell my children all the time that no one can ever come close to the kind of human Mark was. I do not make these kinds of comments usually. He is someone who truly was special. You meet someone like this once in a generation, or once in a lifetime, and I meet hundreds of people. I am one of the busiest doctors in the country."

Dr. John told me he has Mark's picture on his desk, right next to his family photo. He asked Sue how she and Ray could have a child like Mark, and she simply said, "He was Mark. Mark was Mark." We laughed and agreed that Sue doesn't take any credit. "Through all of this, we cannot forget Sue. Mark's story is her story."

"My relationship with Mark was a very special one. It was a unique and long connection for many, many years. It is very hard to do justice to Mark. It had to start with Mark being a very mature, strong-willed child. Strong character coming from a child. Maturity far beyond his years. Add those two together with a heart of gold creates such a combination. Anybody who has

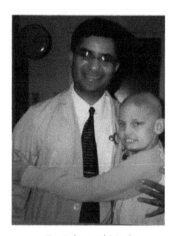
Dr. John and Mark

come across Mark agrees that it was a special encounter."

Mark always hugged Dr. John when saying goodbye. One time, Mark was walking down the hallway and shouted back at Dr. John, "I love you." And Dr. John, without hesitation, shouted back, "I love you too, Mark!"

Dr. John shared one last memory: "One time, I vividly remember, Mark came in and had a treatment. He had been in a great deal of pain and asked to come in and see me. I did something I have never done before. Usually, immediately after the treatment, which only lasted a few minutes, Mark would be out the door." Mark wanted a sandwich, and Sue was going to leave the room and to get one for him.

"We had this time alone. On this day, I told my nurse, 'Take my pager; I do not want to be disturbed.' Mark and I had a conversation and chatted and chatted. I now wish I had done that more often." There was silence for a few seconds, and in this silence, I could feel Dr. John lost in this powerful memory.

"I gained strength from this conversation; I gained strength and inspiration. I don't know why I did this on this day, but the memory still brings a tear to my eye. It was the last time I ever saw Mark."

I asked Dr. John for any closing comments, and after a few minutes of quiet consideration, he said, "You have to put selfless and generous together to speak of Mark's greatness. His suffering was permanent, and so was his kindness."

CHAPTER TWENTY: THE STAEHELY FAMILY

"Dear God, I want to thank you for my Father. Thank you for letting us be together. Thank you for giving him a great job where he can be with me a lot. Thank you for keeping him strong and well enough to do things with me. Finally, thank you for helping us get along. Also, I just want to thank you for a few more things. First of all I want to thank you for my great family. Thank you for letting me spend time with them.

Thank you for keeping them healthy and letting them take care of me. I need you to help my brother get a good job, that he would like and not struggle at. He's a good brother and I would do anything for him, so please keep your eye on him and always protect him. Thank you God. Last, Thanks for giving us all the Power, strength and courage to move on. Finally, please bless all my family and thanks for all your blessings. Amen.

Mark Staehely

This book would not be complete without a chapter about the Staehely family: Ray, Sue, and Michael, better known as "Mark's family."

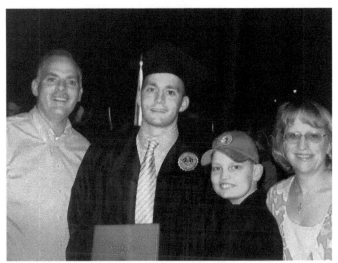

Michael's college graduation

When a family learns their child has cancer, and the prognosis is not good, no one would be surprised if they crept into a place where they were not exposed so that they could process the diagnosis and learn to put one foot in front of the other in private. Not the Staehely family.

From the very beginning, they opened up their home and their hearts to anyone willing to take this journey with them. They never once asked for privacy or to be left alone; this was apparent the night of Mark's diagnosis when they invited family and friends to their home. They embraced the out-pouring of love and support and allowed us to learn from what we have come to know as Mark's greatness.

As previously mentioned, the Staehelys were an ordinary, unpretentious Midwestern family working hard to provide a safe and happy home for their kids. Unremarkable until the unimaginable happened, the family suddenly became exposed to the horrors of cancer and the struggles of living everyday with a sick child.

For those of us who came together to support them, the emotional and financial burden was beyond anything any of us had ever experienced. Family, friends, and community pulled together with fundraisers to offer support. Sue and I began this journey as neighbors, and our friendship has grown into one of my life's greatest treasures.

I have spent endless hours talking, crying, and sharing stories with the Staehelys. We have collaborated on this book, and their support and encouragement has been invaluable. Without their willingness and openness to share Mark with all of us, this book would not have been possible.

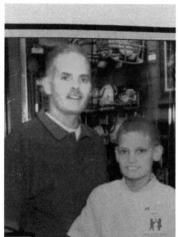
Ray and Mark

One wonders how Mark became this extraordinary child? What was it about his upbringing that brought out his passion for love and his deep need to give back to others? I believe the generosity they showed in sharing Mark with us proves exactly where Mark got his generous spirit. In many conversations with Ray and Sue, I listened carefully for a hint, some advice or words of wisdom on how to raise a child like Mark. But they take very little credit for him.

Ray states, "We learned more from Mark than he ever learned from us." As parents, they feel lucky to have been able to foster Mark's dreams. From the beginning of Mark's illness, they strove to make his life as normal as possible. "Normal" meant being with his friends regardless of his blood counts and susceptibility to infection. It meant riding the four-wheeler or his bike when a simple fall could mean serious injury. Allowing him to live his life the way *he* saw fit meant they were giving him every opportunity. Sue and Ray knew every day was a gift for Mark.

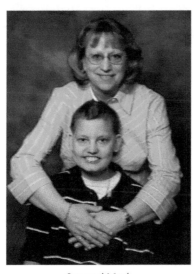

Sue and Mark

Mark loved Sue's cooking. He craved her tomato salad and asked for it often. She cooked anything Mark asked for at any hour of the day. Since Mark didn't sleep very well, Sue often sat up with him. It wasn't unusual for Mark to crave McDonald's French fries in the middle of the night. Sue would dash off to pick them up, only to get home to find he had lost his appetite. Ray explained that if Mark craved a steak, they would hop in the car at any hour and find a place to order a steak for Mark.

Mark often longed for bacon, and Sue bought it in bulk. She said their house constantly smelled of cooked bacon. Smiling, she said, "If Mark ate it, I would cook it, anything to keep weight on him."

Sue and Ray weren't the only members of the household to make changes to accommodate Mark. When his brother was diagnosed, Mike felt there was no question that he would stay close to home and attend Joliet Junior College. Mike was able to spend a lot of time with Mark during those two years, and he cherishes the time they spent together.

Mike reflected on a special memory. It was the second year of Mark's illness, and he was in the hospital for the Fourth of July. Mike did not spend much alone time with Mark, so this was a special time for just the two of them. On this particular day, Mike was staying the night at the hospital with Mark and had an idea. He told Mark, "Hey, we're in downtown Chicago, and it's the Fourth of July. The fireworks are crazy down here. Let's find a place where we can enjoy them." Mike lifted Mark into his wheelchair and set out to find the perfect spot. Knowing they were not allowed but not willing to ask permission, Mike found a way to the rooftop of the hospital. There, they witnessed the most spectacular fireworks show either of them had ever experienced. Every July Fourth, the memory of that night returns, and he tells the story to his children, so they, too, will know their Uncle Mark. His wife, Amanda, never had the opportunity to meet Mark, but she knows all the stories and shares them, along with pictures of Mark, with the children.

To this day, when Mike is having a bad day, the stresses of life seem less significant. Because of Mark, he focuses on family and friends and what is most important. Mark taught Mike many lessons, such as how to find the good in any situation. Mark found ways to improve his life and the lives of those around him. More than anything, Mark wanted to make people happy.

As fall of 2002 approached, Mark got stronger. It looked like he'd be able to go back to school on a limited basis when he felt strong and was not traveling to the city for procedures. Mike, along with his parents, thought it was a good time to pack up and move to Normal to attend Illinois State University. The four of them set out to move Mike into his apartment. After they left for home, he found a note in his desk drawer. It was from Mark, telling him good luck, how much he loved him, and how he would think about him often. He remembered Mark carrying around his spiral notebook, always writing his prayers and special notes to his family and friends.

Mike believes Mark suddenly came into his own after his diagnosis, and his true character burst through the

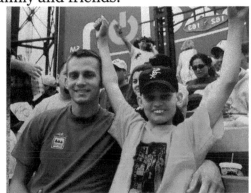

Michael and Mark at a White Sox Game

tough, ornery boy he had once been. He can't explain why but said they never saw the ornery Mark after that. The toughness carried him through his illness, and Mark's caring and loving self genuinely ruled his life.

Michael stated, "Although Mark was unable to get up and move around, he found ways to show us he loved us. Mark never lost his faith. He was aware the odds were stacked against him; he knew better than any of us how sick he was. Through his cancer, Mark found the best of himself."

From the beginning, they knew he would not be around forever. They wanted Mark to have as much quality of life as possible. And that required taking many chances and following Mark's lead on what he could and could not do. Not every day was good, but one day in particular they would always remember.

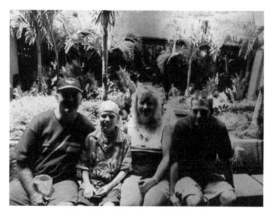

Ray, Sue, Mark and Michael
Hawaii vacation, through Make-A-Wish Foundation

In 2004, Make-A-Wish Foundation granted Mark a wish. Because of his birthday, December 7, he had a special interest in Pearl Harbor. He chose Hawaii, and they were able to visit and fulfill his dream.

From the first day of his diagnosis, when they opened their home to family and friends, until the last week of Mark's life, this family welcomed and embraced the love we all had for Mark.

The Staehely family may not take much credit for the remarkable kid Mark became, but a quote from Sue and Ray will always stay with me: "There was a magnitude of Mark."

Yes, there was...

Chapter Twenty-One: Make Your Mark

*"If you give freely in life from your
heart, it will always come back to you
1000 times over."*

Mark Staehely

Mark believed these words and proved them over and over by his actions. From the many stories I have shared with you, I hope you can feel the heart of this boy. He was wise beyond his years, and to this day, I believe his legacy of giving back carries on in each of us.

Despite the horror of cancer, this family pulled from the magic of Mark and moved forward to accomplish remarkable missions in Mark's honor.

Mark made Sue and Ray promise that they would carry on his toy drive and the search for a cure for neuroblastoma. From these promises, the "Make Your Mark: The Mark Staehely Pediatric Cancer Foundation" was created. It consists of people whom Mark personally asked to be involved; I was lucky enough to be one of them. Over the past eleven years, the foundation has raised over one million dollars! Hundreds of people attend his benefit, years after he has passed away. Some never had the chance to meet him.

Make Your Mark Foundation

Within the foundation, the Mark Staehely Family Assistance Program was developed to help children battling cancer and their families. The Staehely family was well aware of the day-to-day financial struggles a family experiences. Assistance includes items like gas cards, McDonald's food cards, or a cash donation to help with personal needs. The Family Assistance Program is the heart of the foundation.

The Mark Fund at Northwestern Memorial Hospital is an extension of this program. It provides assistance to children who are receiving radiation at Northwestern Memorial and their families. The MARK (My Achievement Recognition Kit) in the Radiation/Oncology department provides a backpack to the patient on their first day of treatment. This kit offers a water bottle, MARK bear, crayons, and bubbles. The parents also receive a packet with $40.00 in meal tickets and five parking vouchers. Upon graduation from radiation, a custom gift is offered to each patient.

A generous donation provided a pediatric waiting room that is located within the larger department waiting room at Northwestern Memorial Hospital. Two iPads are available with different games for patients to enjoy, and the TV streams child-friendly movies throughout the day. There are puzzles, books, and games for a variety of age levels. Mark loved to draw and sketch, and his artwork of a butterfly was enlarged and made into wall decals. In addition to the "Mark a Great Day" wall and waiting room, an exam room was dedicated to pediatrics for follow-up appointments and consultations.

The Foundation has given thousands of dollars to Dr. Mary Beth Madonna at Ann & Robert H. Lurie Children's Hospital and Dr. John Kalapurakal at Northwestern Memorial Hospital for research in neuroblastoma.

Dr. Susan Cohen from Comer Children's Hospital at the University of Chicago is the latest recipient of a Make Your Mark Research Grant. The news is encouraging in the research for a cure for neuroblastoma, but we still need much work and support.

Every April, the Foundation supports a three-day oncology day camp program in downtown Chicago. In 1978, Dr. Edward Barum, a pediatric oncologist at Children's Memorial Hospital in Chicago, had an idea. He understood the social challenges sick children face and the many missed school and social activities they miss out on while being ill. In response, the One Step at a Time Summer Camp was developed.

Campers can experience the fun of the One-Step program while still sleeping in their own beds at night. Activities include a trip to the Chicago Children's Museum, Shedd Aquarium, and other city favorite features. Today the One-Step program has extended beyond summer and includes horseback riding, skiing, educational, and urban camps serving kids from Chicagoland and neighboring communities.

One of the most significant accomplishments of the Foundation is the Mark Staehely Fellowship Award in Oncology and Stem Cell Transplant at Lurie's Children's Hospital.

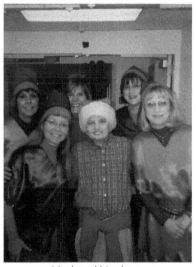

Mark and his elves

Established in 2007, it supports a fellow in oncology and stem cell transplant. The fellowship was fully endowed and will support it for eternity. The Mark Staehely Fellowship Award ensures a sustainable future for the future oncologists at Lurie Children's.

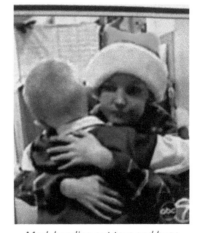
Mark's elves continuing the toy drive

The toy drive began as a family project separate from the Foundation as its heart lies with Ray and Sue. There is a Treasure Chest Program in three different hospitals: Lurie Children's Hospital, Northwestern University Hospital in Chicago, and Presence St. Joseph Hospital in Joliet, Illinois. There is a toy chest on each pediatric floor that provides a small toy for a child who needs a procedure or who is having a bad day. This program continues year-round.

Mark handing out toys and hugs

For a few years, the Foundation supported a scholarship program for young men or women pursuing a degree in fire science. After anonymous nominations, the Board would vote on the recipient. Our son Alex was the recipient one year, and we believe Mark walks beside Alex in his career as a firefighter/paramedic.

During the most challenging years of their lives, this family continued Mark's legacy of giving back. Their grace, sense of community, and generous hearts make it clear how this young boy grew into such an extraordinary young man. Because of their generosity, we were all changed.

(Author's note: Contact information for Make Your Mark: The Mark Staehely Pediatric Cancer Foundation is available at the end of this book.)

CHAPTER TWENTY-TWO: THE BEST YEAR

*"Dear God. Thank you so much for my
scans coming out all clear. I knew I
could do it. But that was a miracle but I
need another miracle, please make my
counts go up. That would be wonderful.
I love you lord. Amen."*

Mark Staehely

2002-2003

In the summer of 2002, Mark was gaining weight, his hair was growing back, and although they hesitated to speak of remission, Mark showed signs of improvement. He was tolerating his medications orally, and his doctors decided to remove his PICC line.

The boys spent endless hours swimming in our pool or at JP and Jonathan's. Mark had a new freedom, and he was not going to waste a single minute.

One afternoon, Mark and Alex wanted to ride the four-wheeler that had gathered dust in the garage. Sue allowed them to ride it in our

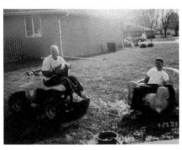

The boys on the four-wheeler

backyards with strict orders to be careful. The boys asked if they could get the hose out and make some puddles; we said yes as we didn't see any harm in a few puddles of water. We were not paying close attention, and before we knew it, they had made a small pond right between our yards. The four-wheeler and the boys were splattered in grass and mud from head to toe. The once-manicured lawns, full of ruts with muddy tire marks throughout, were quite a sight to see. The boys splashed and laughed, and the messier it became, the happier they were.

Ray and my husband Dave arrived home from work to find their once beautiful yards ripped to pieces. Seeing the faces of these boys quickly diminished their shock and horror at the destroyed yards. Grass grows back; memories last a lifetime.

August 21, 2002, was the first day of school. Mark and Alex stood on the curb, waiting for the bus while Sue and I watched from our front windows. It had been two years since Mark had attended classes. Working closely with the principal at Troy Junior High, Mark was allowed to start attending eighth grade with Alex.

Bonfires, basement parties, and school dances: these everyday teenage events consumed their time. Mark attended every sporting event possible and always cheered the loudest.

January 2003

I invited Sue and Mark to join Alex and me at Starved Rock State Park in Utica, Illinois. As a family, we had spent many Labor Day weekends there. The facility has an indoor pool, a warm and cozy great room, and beautiful grounds surrounded by miles and miles of woods. Because weekends at this popular state park book months in advance, we chose January 28, 2003, a weeknight, allowing the boys to miss a day of school.

The boys arrived home from school and were anxious and excited. Heavy snow had been piling up all day. By the time they walked in the door from school, several inches of snow had accumulated. Determined, we packed the car and set out on our journey. The roads were horrible, and the snow wasn't letting up. Sue and I both knew we should cancel, but neither of us had the heart to do so. The one-hour drive took nearly two. It was slow and treacherous. We arrived late but safe.

We had dinner in the lodge, but the boys barely ate a bite because they were anxious to swim. In the pool, Mark jumped off Alex's shoulders over and over as the sounds of laughter echoed off the walls. They were as loud and rowdy

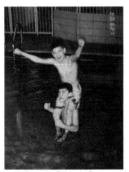

as any two teenagers could be. They had the entire facility to themselves and spent hours splashing in the pool and hot tub, loving every minute. Sue

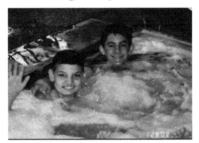

Mark and Alex enjoying the pool

and I relaxed as we listened to their loud laughter and watched the snow continuing to fall outside the warmth of the lodge. On this one night, life was normal, and Mark was living in the moment; on this bitter, snowy winter night, all we felt was warmth and contentment.

The boys stayed up late watching movies. The next day we woke up to a bright, sunny day, a perfect winter wonderland. The trees were laced with snow, and the snowdrifts piled five feet high.

Hiking was out of the question, so we decided to drive around the park and enjoy the landscape as much as we could from the warmth of our car. As we drove down by the Illinois River, we saw other cars stopped, and people were getting out, walking toward the river. Luckily, the road and parking lot had recently been plowed.

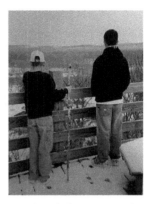

Mark and Alex at Starved Rock

Unable to see beyond the road, we parked and walked down toward the river. As we stood there, we saw a bald eagle fly right over us. As if for our very own personal pleasure, the eagle landed, and another joined it. They sat there in all their glory as if to welcome us to the day, and to create a memory that would last forever.

(Author's note: Sixteen years later, I have returned to Starved Rock alone. After three years of seriously writing this book, I have struggled with these last three chapters and felt a pull here. As I sat down and opened my laptop, I felt a sense of calm and focus. I wrote for three hours before I realized my back was aching, and I needed to stretch. I left my room and went for a walk. When I returned, my mind was full of words and inspiration empowered me.)

March 2003 - Rocky

Mark was an animal lover, unlike his mom. He had begged for a dog from the time he was old enough to talk, but the answer had always been no. Then our family got a new puppy, Josie. Mark fell in love with her and spent as much time as he could, loving and playing with her.

One day, I heard about a puppy who looked just like our Josie, a little black and white Shih Tzu. Catching Ray and Sue in a weak moment, I showed them the picture of the adorable puppy. Looking so much like our Josie, they agreed Mark could have him. We decided to make it a surprise for Mark. Needing an extra set of hands, I invited my girlfriend Jill to go with me to pick up the puppy. We bought a crate, dog food, toys, and everything else they would need to welcome him home.

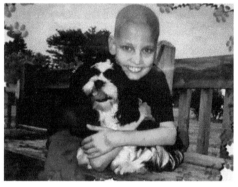

Mark and his beloved Rocky

After a long day at the hospital, Mark returned home, and Alex called him to see if he felt like coming over. It didn't take long for Mark to show up, and with Sue and Ray sneaking in the back door, we brought the little guy to Mark. His face, full of shock and disbelief, turned into a wide grin, and his eyes sparkled and filled with tears, realizing the dog belonged to him. I'm not sure who was more excited, Mark or the puppy; both were jumping and racing around the room. This day will be forever etched in my mind. Mark, beaming with joyful tears, named him Rocky, and they were inseparable.

Mark's attendance in classes was sporadic at best. His doctor and hospital visits continued, and it wasn't long before he had the port inserted again to receive much-needed blood and platelets.

Mark began chemotherapy on a maintenance program. Once again, he lost his hair but maintained his stamina and stayed involved in extracurricular activities. Mark, being Mark, had become the center of his peers. They included Mark in everything, and when the eighth-grade dance approached, Mark knew what he wanted to do. He had a few contacts and planned a big surprise for his friends.

The night arrived, and the group of sixteen kids met at the Staehely house for pictures. Pulling

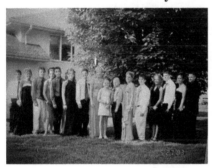

up to the curb was a fancy, white stretch limousine! One of Mark's special friends had made a kind gesture, donating the limo for the evening, full of sparkling water for all the kids.

The eighth grade dance attendees

Following the dance, they were picked up by their driver and completed their evening in style. The evening was magical, and if there had been a king of the night's festivities, Mark would have worn the crown proudly.

Graduation Class 2002-2003

There was never a question that Mark would be allowed to graduate with his friends. Troy School District had supported Mark for three years and gave him the credit they felt he deserved. In their view, his diploma had been earned, and he was entitled to walk across that stage.

Mark stood tall and proud as he crossed the stage in his blue cap and gown. The presenter boldly announced, "Mark Staehely."

The gym grew quiet, and all eyes were on Mark. He approached Mr. Wiers and reached his hand out to accept his diploma. As he did, he smiled and looked up at Mr. Wiers, saying, "I love you; don't ever give up." The entire audience in the gymnasium offered a standing ovation for Mark. This ceremony was a moment of profound accomplishment for Mark, and the audience shared a sense of pride for a young man who not only persevered but also made his "Mark" on the students and staff at Troy Middle School.

Together, we all joined to celebrate Mark's presence and the friendships he had formed with the class of 2002-2003. Mark, the teacher and mentor. Mark, our hero.

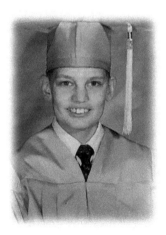

"A true friend reaches for your hand and touches your heart."
Anonymous

CHAPTER TWENTY-THREE: THE FINAL CHAPTER

"I've seen heaven and I've seen God."

Mark Staehely

In 2004, Mark became involved with our local Hospice Chapter as a volunteer. After a few weeks, he asked his Hospice nurse if he could work for her. Especially for Mark, she created an "Executive Assistant" position. He decided he wanted to earn and save money to buy his own sports cards for his favorite hobby.

Hospice took over Mark's pain management and this cut down on many trips to the city. His nurse and "boss," Kim, remembered how Mark began his two-hour shift walking around and charming all the ladies in the office. He was a hard worker (when he wasn't socializing) and took great pride in the jobs she gave him. After working only a month, Mark decided to ask for a raise. With that grin and self-confidence, he walked into the office of the CEO and walked out with a raise and a smile that matched his pride.

One of Mark's favorite jobs was grading papers for tests that had been given to the staff. Sue said Mark's favorite part was using the red pen!

Mark knew significant sadness in his young life. He made deep friendships while a patient at the hospital, and during his six years of illness he suffered many losses. Don Cameron, his beloved friend and a Make Your Mark board member, passed away in 2004. Working for Hospice was a great source of support for him.

One day Sue went to pick up Mark. He was still busy with his work, and without looking up from his paper, he quietly said, "I've seen Heaven, and I've seen God." Everyone stopped what they were doing, and a sudden hush and stillness filled the room.

Sue said, "You've seen what?"

He repeated, "I've seen Heaven, and I've seen God."

Sue asked him, "What does God look like?"

Again, without taking his eyes off the paper, he replied, "He looks just like His pictures, of course."

A few minutes later, he commented on the beauty of heaven and the flowers there. He said, "What a glorious place." He talked about his friend Don who had died.

Softly, he said, "I am not afraid to die. I know Heaven is home."

The next few days became excruciating for Mark. His beloved Hospice volunteers, with whom he'd grown so close, were always on call. Sue and Ray struggled with taking him back to the hospital, but it was extremely painful for Mark to move or be touched.

Sue had never wanted Mark to die at home, but she and Ray realized transferring Mark would be unbearable and confided their concerns in one of Mark's favorite nurses from Children's and closest friends, Jane, who was a constant support. Together, they controlled his pain and made him as comfortable as possible. He could stay surrounded by everyone and everything he loved.

As difficult as it was, they decided to put a hospital bed in the family room and let Hospice take over his care. Mark was aware of this decision, and he agreed he wanted to stay home.

One day he asked Sue, "What day is it?" She replied, "March third." He just nodded his head.

Sue and Ray generously opened their home to anyone who wanted to visit Mark. Dozens and dozens of people came and went that week. JP, Alex, and Jonathan were with him every chance they had throughout the week.

A couple of days later, Mark again asked Sue for the date.

She replied, "March sixth. Why, Mark? Why do you keep asking?"

He didn't answer. Suddenly it hit Sue, and she said to Ray, "Mark is waiting until March seventh." His favorite number seven!

She knew without a doubt that Mark only had one more day.

Gradually, they had to increase his medication to ease the intense pain he was experiencing. Mark wanted to talk to everyone, as he always was the talker, and wanted to be aware of his surroundings. In Mark fashion, each and every visitor was given the signature "I love you" before they left.

Those of us who visited were in awe of this incredible gesture, opening their home in their child's final days, that Sue and Ray demonstrated. We were aware we were saying goodbye, aware our presence took away from their own precious time with Mark. This selfless act on their part allowed us the opportunity to process our own depth of loss, together with Mark. Some people stayed only a few minutes; others remained for hours. Sue, Ray, and Michael were always close by.

Sue called me at work to tell me Mark's time was near, and I immediately drove home. She invited me to come over and invited the boys. I called Adam at NIU, and he was in Shorewood in record time.

I expected to feel an overwhelming sadness and dread, but when I walked into the house, I heard laughter and conversation. The house was abuzz. Hospice explained to us that even if Mark appeared asleep, he could still hear us and was aware of our presence. It was a bit more subdued in the family room where Mark lay snuggled under layers of blankets, but what I felt was a kind of comfort and closeness. Mark and I had our time together, mostly in silence, holding hands. We shared our "love yous."

The truth is there are no words to describe that moment, the moment when I realized I would never again see his broad smile or hear his distinctive laugh.

Slowly, peacefully, Mark slipped into unconsciousness. Mark took his last breath in the family room of their home, the same place where he'd watched hundreds of baseball games with his dad and brother, snuggled with his mom, and spent hours on the computer.

It was March 7th, six days after Mark had told his mother he wasn't afraid to die because he knew heaven was home. Surrounded by dozens of family and friends, Mark quietly and peacefully went home.

The funeral home came to the house, and we all went outside to give the family some peace and privacy. As they brought Mark out the front door, we stood on the sidewalk, joined together, holding hands. In the warmth of the sunshine, there was total silence as we bowed our heads. I still see us there, feel that warm silence almost every day. What we knew in that moment is that we had shared the gift of Mark. Because of Mark, we would never be the same. We were better people, kinder and more generous. We had learned from an extraordinary human being. Mark's life meant something. His example of loving others was as if he were a living angel, full of life lessons and grace.

And it wasn't just those of us who saw him every day who felt his impact. The Troy Fire Department respectfully gave Mark a full Honor Guard service at his funeral.

Mark's faith was not just something he wrote about; it was something he believed and lived with every ounce of his being.

CHAPTER TWENTY-FOUR: THE DIME

*"I can feel my loved ones standing right
beside me in every challenge I face."*

Mark Staehely

"If only we had a dime for every time we
drove up here, Mark." Sue and Ray must have said
that dozens of times over the six years of Mark's
illness. Little did they or anyone understand the
significance of dimes in the years that would follow
Mark's death.

There are several meanings regarding the
finding of dimes:

- A message from above

- Ancestors, spirits, guides, or deceased
loved ones want you to know they are
looking out for you

- The number ten symbolizes a circle,
coming full circle, fulfillment, unity, or
completion

- Guidance or validation that you are in
the right place

- A reminder that you are loved and
valued

- A sign that positive changes are on their
way

- A reward or token of approval from
beyond

- Someone or something is trying to get
your attention

The first dime showed up the day Mark passed away. Ray, needing to get away by himself, decided to take a walk around the yard, his domain and personal space. With a heart full of resignation, he felt powerless over the present and unsure about the future. He did not notice the early signs of spring or if the grass needed to be cut.

As Ray approached the sidewalk, something caught his eye: a bright, shiny dime. No one else had noticed it as they stood together. Ray picked it up without thinking and walked into a now quiet and practically empty house. Only Sue and Michael remained. He showed it to them. Immediately Sue said, "Well, that's obviously from Mark."

Weeks later, as I was getting dressed to attend the first Make Your Mark Foundation board meeting, I walked downstairs to the laundry room in my robe. I saw a dime on the stairs and reached down to put it in my pocket without giving it another thought. I felt something else in my pocket and pulled out another dime. Thinking it odd but not noteworthy, I put them on the kitchen counter.

Later that morning, at the meeting, Sue shared Ray's story. I felt goosebumps and a sudden rush of excitement. It hit me: What was a dime doing in my robe? Who puts money in a robe? I told my dime story to the group, and that became the first of many stories the dime has produced.

Over the past few years, I've found many dimes. Following my interview with Larry Wiers, I walked to my car, and as I looked down to open the door, a dime flashed up at me. I pictured Mark smiling down on us for spending two hours talking solely about him.

I don't question their appearance; I stop, pick them up, take a deep breath, and smile. I've shared my dime story many times with people, and it is nothing short of amazing when I run into someone with a dime story of their own to share with me.

Be prepared; once you've heard these stories about the significance of dimes, you will find one at a particular time that is unique to you, and that dime will take on new meaning.

Our son Adam was on his way to Lurie Children's Hospital to visit a close family friend of ours whose eight-month-old daughter had been diagnosed with leukemia that morning. Walking in a daze of shock and worry, he glanced down as the elevator door opened. There was a dime. He bent down, picked it up, and put it in his pocket. When he reached the hospital room, he handed the dime to his friend and told her the story. There was hope in that moment. Today that beautiful little champion is in total remission.

Last year, Christine had a secret Santa gift to buy for a teen boy. Not familiar with teen boy interests, she struggled to find the right gift. On Mark's birthday, December 7th, she was out shopping for the perfect gift. The boy had an interest in arts. She glanced down, and right on the sidewalk outside the arts and crafts shop was a shiny dime. Her task suddenly became an unexpected joy from Mark and reassurance that art supplies would be a perfect gift for this boy.

Jonathan remembers that after Mark's death, he started to find a lot of dimes. Dimes became a sign to him that Mark was watching over him. He told me he has randomly found a dime when he is having a bad day, needs courage for something, or is about to do something exciting.

Since becoming a fireman, Alex tucks a dime in his helmet and jacket, and he carries it with him on every call.

Regardless of your faith, the dime is a physical and substantial reminder that Mark is still working, sharing his humor and his gifts.

Mark, funny and friendly, taught hundreds of people that the simple act of giving back is the greatest act of kindness in the world—giving of your talents, your money, and your loving spirit to those who are willing to accept it.

Mark's life was too short but well lived. His many lessons can bring us hope and encouragement, one shiny dime at a time.

~THE MEMORY GARDEN~

The summer after Mark passed away, Sue and Ray decided to create a memory garden in their backyard. Many people participated in the design and digging of the garden. It was a labor of love.

They chose a variety of flowers. There were petunias, geraniums, and dozens of perennials that filled the garden with bursts of color. Year after year Sue picks different varieties, and Ray lovingly digs and turns the soil to prepare the garden.

A wooden bench placed in the center provides a quiet place to sit and remember. As you walk or drive by their house, it is easily seen from the street, and you can't help but take notice as it invites you to visit.

Luckily for me, I see this garden every day. Often, I walk over to the garden, holding the tiny hand of my granddaughter. As we walk up to the garden, I take a deep breath and tell her about Mark, the boy next door.

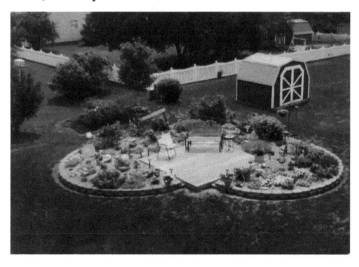

Remember Me

Remember me, he said one day.
Please don't forget, I cannot stay.
I have to leave, I will not heal.
Remember me; this is for real.

My cancer won't go, I cannot stay.
I fought so hard for one more day.
Don't stop the fight to find a cure.
I'll watch and help, you can be sure.

Learn from me, I tried to teach
each of you to always reach
For one more dream, for one more way
to make a difference, every day.

Time is short, yes, I am proof
that some die young and leave too soon.
Please take the time, I never had...
To change the world, like I would have.

Always please
Remember me

by Peggy Lindgren

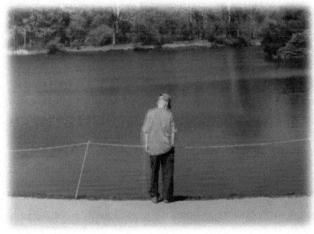

~ ACKNOWLEDGEMENTS ~

I want to thank my husband, Dave, for his love,
reassurance, and understanding when I was so
engrossed in writing that I pretended I didn't know he
was standing right behind me. Also, for helping me
with many computer issues!

I appreciate Adam, Sarah, Alex, and Shelly for their
love, advice, and encouragement during the last
several years of this project.

To my best girlfriends and sisters: You know who you
are. I thank you for your amazing friendships and for
the many toasts you made on my behalf!

To my Yorkville Writers Group and to Lisa, our
facilitator, for being the ones who made this book a
reality, I sincerely thank you for having confidence in
me when I was uncertain I could move forward and for
your excellent critiques month after month. I value
your friendships. Especially to Anne, for inviting me to
this group and for her extra editing skills and advice.
Also, for writing the forward to this book.

Thank you to each of you who contributed your
personal stories about Mark and for your willingness
to share them with others. Your stories were exactly
why I felt Mark's story needed to be told. The many
lives he touched went far beyond my own. I only wish I
could have included more of those stories.

I especially offer my heartfelt appreciation to Ray, Sue,
and Michael for their constant support. Your faith in
me to write Mark's story has been an honor and a
privilege. Thank you for the many hours of
conversation and reminiscence. I also appreciate your
patience.

~ About The Author ~

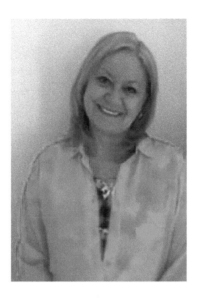

Peggy Lindgren is a wife, mother, and grandmother. She enjoys gardening, traveling, and her Four Seasons Book Club.

She has been a member of the Yorkville Adult Writers Group for over three years and credits them for helping her fulfill her dream.

Although she has written articles for an online website and the local newspaper, this is her first published book.

When it came to writing this memoir, she knew it would be a challenge, an emotional journey that was years in the making. Mark's story has always been in her heart, and her vision was to share his legacy.

Make Your Mark: The Mark Staehely Pediatric Cancer Foundation continues to work to make a difference in the lives of children living with pediatric cancers.

If you are interested in learning more about Make Your Mark: The Mark Staehely Pediatric Cancer Foundation, visit makeyourmark7.org

CPSIA information can be obtained
at www.ICGtesting.com
Printed in the USA
LVHW010840040820
662306LV00011B/744